LOW
BLOOD
SUGAR

LOW BLOOD SUGAR

Peter J. Steincrohn, M.D.

HENRY REGNERY COMPANY • Chicago

FOR

Patti, Barbara, Alan, Joel,
Jennifer, Dorothy, Dave, Nancy, Dan, Jeffrey
— who know (or will grow up to know)
why they are a part of this dedication.

Contents

All letters and case histories cited
are from the author's files.
Names and initials have been changed to
protect private identities.

Note

Doctor Steincrohn, we who suffer from hypoglycemia have no bread except gluten or high protein bread—and only one or two slices daily. We take few starches, no refined sugar in any form, and no caffeine—which eliminates chocolate, cola drinks, and regular coffee.

Admittedly, this may be an expensive and monotonous diet, but along with taking adrenal cortex extract it keeps us well. Diet is the more important part of the treatment.

Millions of us have gone from doctor to doctor, seeking relief from our miseries, only to be told we are suffering from acute anxiety. Or we are given tranquilizers and sent to psychiatrists.

I suffered from nearly all of the unpleasant symptoms: dizziness, fear, panic, chronic exhaustion, compulsive eating and drinking, antisocial behavior, blurred vision, hysteria, suicidal tendencies. Lack of proper attention to this disease ruined all my young years.

Then I found an internist who had done his homework. After three weeks of a special diet and injections, I was a new woman at 48. I began really to live for the first time. You have no idea what it means to be able to say that.

If doctors had bothered to give me the six-hour glucose tolerance test many years ago, I wouldn't have lost so much of my life.

I believe that hypoglycemia causes broken homes, contributes to juvenile delinquency, drug addiction, suicide, alcoholism, and mental confusion. Thousands are desperate today because hypoglycemia has not been recognized.

I am so grateful to my doctor. I've lost forty pounds, have a good job, and have married again. For the first time in my life, I am truly happy.

In my opinion, the six-hour glucose tolerance test should be mandatory in all mental institutions, jails, prisons, juvenile halls, and in any other places where disturbed or troublesome persons are being held.

I hope, Dr. Steincrohn, that you keep emphasizing the importance of testing for low blood sugar. Many readers will recognize these symptoms as their own or those of someone they know.

As a favor to me, and to the many thousands who now need it more than I do, please put it all into a book.

Mrs. C.

Thanks, Mrs. C. I agree. Proof? Here's my book.

P. J. S.

Introduction

You may not actually feel sick; nevertheless, you say, "I don't know what it is, but I could feel better." Perhaps you suffer from the "nervous housewife syndrome." Or in midafternoons you take aspirin for "executive headache."

You cannot understand why you fade so easily. So many of your friends have greater responsibilities than you have; yet they never complain of fatigue or exhaustion. Their children are a pleasure rather than trial; their jobs are a pleasant challenge rather than a daily threat to their very existence. If you work in an office, do you begin, around 3 P.M., to fight the hands of the clock, wondering how you will withstand the torture of trying to stay awake and alert for two more devastating hours?

You're not sick. The doctor says so. Yet you're not well. "There must be something wrong somewhere," you say to yourself. But where? Has the doctor overlooked the trouble? It's possible. Let me put it more succinctly: it's likely!

1

As an internist, I know that most patients who come in for a complete physical checkup do not have a special examination called a blood sugar tolerance test. Only when diabetes is suspected does one usually have the benefit of such an examination.

And thereby hangs the tale. Hundreds of thousands of innocent, unsuspecting Americans drag themselves through their trying days, unaware that they are suffering from the "hunger disease"—from sugar starvation. Their muscles, their brains, their livers, are frantically asking for more sugar in the blood to give them energy and strength to live at optimum efficiency. It is undoubtedly true that many more people suffer from *hypoglycemia* (low blood sugar) than from *hyperglycemia* (high blood sugar)—as in diabetes mellitus.

If your pancreas is secreting too much insulin and you are unaware that you are suffering from hyperinsulinism and resulting hypoglycemia, you are the victim of an overlooked diagnosis. I believe that no medical examination can be considered complete without proper blood sugar determinations. These are as essential in diagnosis as blood pressure readings, stethoscopic examinations, electrocardiograms, and X rays. It is because these relatively simple blood studies are not made that you may forever drag yourself through endless days of misery rather than skip through life. It is ironic to feel ill when you are blessed with an otherwise healthy machine.

Are you supposed to have a borderline case of hypothyroidism? Maybe you are taking thyroid extract but still surrender to daily exhaustion. You and your doctor are nonplussed. Perhaps you are starved for sugar in your blood. Hypoglycemia is a common, though often overlooked, cause of fatigue.

Has your memory been failing lately? Suspicions run through your mind that your brain arteries are hardening and making you prematurely old. It's possible. But, in fact, your healthy arteries and perfectly normal brain cells may not be functioning normally because they are sugar-starved.

Many people have difficulty in staying awake. Are you always sleepy? Is a good night's sleep ineffective in keeping you awake and alert during the day? Perhaps you suffer from narcolepsy, so often associated with hyperinsulinism and low blood sugar. Early diagnosis and treatment can transform your sluggishness into a zestful personality.

Sudden bouts of rapid heart action, sweats, and apprehension make many people believe they are having repeated heart attacks. Does such anxiety for you translate itself into fear of sudden death? Low blood sugar may be the answer. If so, your attacks of despair and fearfulness will probably disappear with treatment.

Are you under treatment by a psychiatrist because of personality changes or because of vague anxieties you cannot account for? Perhaps you, too, are an innocent victim of hypoglycemia. Proper diagnosis and treatment may save you from a protracted course of sessions on the couch (or in the chair) of a psychiatrist.

Mind you, I make no indiscriminate promises. I do not say that recognition and treatment of blood sugar deficiency is the cure-all and catchall for every symptom and disease known to man. But I do insist that too many suffer needlessly because hypoglycemia is too often unrecognized.

I propose to save you from yourself for yourself. Your own doctor will have a hand in it, but your own cooperation will be essential for success. I can show you how to help yourself. I will tell you about special diets and medicines. What to do and what not to do. When and how to alert your doctor to the need for blood sugar tolerance examinations.

If you haven't been feeling up to par for years, and hypoglycemia is the reason, then this book can help you look forward to each new day with happy anticipation rather than remain blanketed by anxiety and deadening fatigue.

There is a solution to your problem: *stop suffering sugar starvation.*

1

The Wanderers

I CALL it the medical merry-go-round.

I see uncomfortable, sugar-starved patients making their weary rounds of physicians' offices; wanderers, hoping to discover at least one who will bring them magical relief, as if they are reaching for the brass ring. Round and round they go. So many, actually dizzy and frustrated in their search for *the* physician who will not fail them.

You might think they should be happy instead of dejected, for doctor after doctor has assured them, "You are all right. I can't find anything wrong with you." Instead of accepting this verdict with relief, they run their fingers down the *Yellow Pages* in search of another medical opinion and another ride on the merry-go-round.

It is possible that you suffer from low blood sugar. And I mean *suffer*. Millions of Americans do. But while they are plagued by discomforting symptoms, they may be treated for something else: anxiety state, hypothyroidism, heart disease, ulcers, migraine, narcolepsy, hysteria, "nervous breakdown."

Case Histories

Two examples illustrate this point.

"For several years I had difficulty in concentrating. Sitting on the bench had become a trying ordeal. I'd get confused and drowsy. When I'd get to the point where I'd feel trembly, I'd order a temporary recess and drink a Coke or munch on a candy bar. I'd come back feeling better, but I'd soon feel worse than I did before.

"Not until a doctor suggested that I might have hypoglycemia did I have a glucose tolerance test. Sure enough, I'd been suffering from low blood sugar. With proper treatment, I feel like a new man. I'm as fresh and alert at the end of the day as I was when I was a youngster."

"I had been so anxious about myself, especially about heart disease because my heart palpitated so much. It seemed to run away with itself. I also had bad migraine headaches. I was extremely restless. You can understand why my family and my many doctors must have regarded me a hopeless hypochondriac—but never said so to my face.

"At last I went to an internist who insisted, against my wishes, that I have a glucose tolerance test. He discovered that I have a low blood sugar curve. After following special diets for a month, my headaches, heart palpitations, and nervousness magically disappeared. My family can't get over this transformation. Neither can I."

And so go the histories of millions of misdiagnosed or undiagnosed cases. One estimate is that 2.5 million Americans suffer from *diabetes mellitus* (too much sugar in the blood). Another conservative estimate is that at least 5 million suffer from the symptoms of *hypoglycemia* (too little sugar in the blood).

For example, a young architect complains of hunger pains two hours after meals—pains relieved by taking food. It seems to be the typical case of duodenal ulcer. Yet his doctor can't find the X-ray changes he expects. Furthermore, continued treatment for duodenal ulcer does not bring improvement.

(Reason? His symptoms are really due to hypoglycemia.)

A young woman is classified as a hopeless neurotic. She is treated for a chronic anxiety state. She trembles and shakes. She has all kinds of fears of impending doom; yet she says, "I can't understand it. There's no earthly reason why I should worry. I have a wonderful husband and fine children. We have no financial worries. Why should I be so nervous?"

(Reason? Undiagnosed hypoglycemia.)

Hypoglycemia is a great simulator. But please don't misunderstand me. I do not offer the diagnosis of low blood sugar as a panacea for all ills and for all patients—a catchall for everything that ails mankind. All I am suggesting is that if you or your doctor are in any doubt whatever about the origin of your complaints, or concerned about lack of response to treatment, you deserve a thorough analysis of your blood sugar content. This is commonly known as the glucose tolerance test.

The Sugar Curve

To understand the problem, you should know the fundamentals of sugar testing. Normally, the fasting blood sugar is anywhere from 65 to 120 mg. (milligrams) per 100 ml. (milliliters) of blood. After a meal, the blood sugar may rise to about 140. When it gets to 170 (and higher), it is definitely above normal, as in diabetic patients. Another abnormality in blood sugar content is the opposite of diabetes: the blood sugar falls too low. This is called hypoglycemia, as distinct from the hyperglycemia of diabetes.

How is the usual blood sugar tolerance curve estimated? You fast for at least twelve hours; then a blood sample is taken from a vein. After the blood is examined for *fasting blood sugar*, you are given a measured amount of sugar solution to drink. Every hour thereafter (for five or six hours) a specimen is taken and examined for sugar content. Meanwhile, you do not eat or drink anything.

Figure A: Normal Sugar Curves

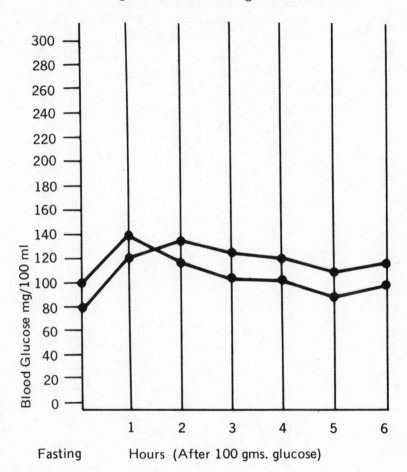

These figures are put down on a chart and connected to reveal the blood sugar curve. (See Figure A.) It is important that at least a five-hour curve be taken, for in some patients the blood sugar may be normal for the first three hours and abruptly drop after four or five hours. If only a three-hour curve is taken, the diagnosis of hypoglycemia may be missed. The reading may be a normal 70 or 80 at the third hour but fall abnormally to a low 40 or 50 in the fifth or sixth hour. (See Figure B.)

Figure B: Hypoglycemic Curves

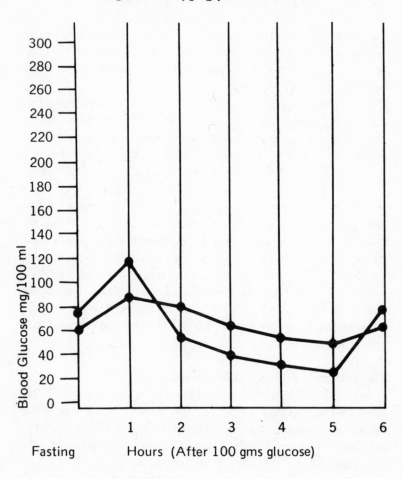

Now suppose the blood sugar curve is abnormally low. What happens? The brain commonly is a target. Since it depends so much on blood sugar for its food and oxygen, it cannot absorb oxygen without the presence of sufficient sugar in the blood. Thus the inefficiency of the brain cells causes the hypoglycemic patient to complain of being jittery, nervous, anxious, restless, confused, drowsy, and, in the most severe cases, actually unconscious. His brain is rebelling against sugar hunger.

Low blood sugar causes fatigue because of lessened sugar supply to muscles. It resembles ulcer hunger pains (as in the architect's case) because the stomach resents the low sugar. It may be mistaken for hypothyroidism because low blood sugar sometimes causes slow reactions and sleepiness.

Consider the traveling salesman who miraculously escaped several near-fatal auto accidents while driving around the state. His trouble was caused by drowsiness at the wheel. He drank coffee and took stay-awake pills, but nothing seemed to help. One day his doctor said, "Let's take a blood sugar tolerance test." He found that the patient had an abnormally low blood sugar. After treatment (which I shall explain later) he no longer felt so drowsy. He hasn't had an accident since.

Hypoglycemia—Cause and Prevention

What causes hypoglycemia? How can we prevent it? These are two large question marks. Most patients have low blood sugar of unknown origin (idiopathic hypoglycemia). Some relatively rare cases are caused by an *islet tumor* in the pancreas. When this tumor is surgically removed, the patient reverts to normal. What we do know is that the pancreas is the organ that secretes insulin, whose job is to burn sugar; we also know that sometimes it oversecretes to cause low blood sugar.

The liver is involved, too. Its job in sugar metabolism is to store unused sugar as *glycogen*. When some upset occurs in storage and liberation of glycogen as sugar usable by the body (sometimes the glandular system is at fault), then the patient may have *hyperinsulinism*—another form of hypoglycemia. (More about the physiology of sugar metabolism in Chapter 2.)

By now I hope you realize' that low blood sugar is no joke. It should not be minimized, especially when it causes symptoms that you or your doctor may mistake for duodenal ulcer, migraine, heart disease, hysteria, anxiety state, or, as one patient said, "simply acting like a lowdown hypochondriac." Nobody likes to wear false labels or to be treated for something he hasn't got. As I'll say here quite often, correct diagnosis is vital but treatment is equally important once the diagnosis has been made.

You go to your doctor. He practices heads-up medicine. He becomes suspicious early, and advises that you come in for a six-hour glucose tolerance test because he believes that low blood sugar is causing your symptoms.

In treatment he will reverse what most people think: instead of ordering you to take sweets to "bring up" your blood sugar, he will advise you to eliminate sweets from your diet. Although a chocolate candy, for instance, may make you feel better for a few minutes because it raises your blood sugar, you will feel worse after it. Why? Because the pancreas will secrete too much insulin to take care of the sugar in the chocolate, and your blood sugar will drop even lower than it was before you ate it.

Your doctor will say, "No candy, cake, pies, ice cream, cookies, sodas." Instead of a high carbohydrate diet, you will need to take a high protein diet. Although some part of this is eventually broken down to sugar, this process is so slow that it does not cause the pancreas to pour out large amounts of insulin.

You will be surprised how you can learn to do without sweets. A high protein diet (meats, fish, fowl, dairy products, cereals) sticks to the ribs. Within a month or two on this rather simple treatment, you will say, if you are a typical hypoglycemic, "It's a miraculous transformation. I haven't felt so good in years."

Remember, however, what I said previously. Such a treatment isn't a catchall cure for all symptoms and all diseases; it is helpful only if no doubt exists about the diagnosis of hypoglycemia.

A Few Practical Tips

Here are a few preliminary tips, to be enlarged on later, for the management of low blood sugar.

1.　*Eat frequently.*　Get into the habit of taking a snack (a glass of milk, a handful of nuts, a piece of cheese) between meals. Also take a snack every two hours before bedtime, following your evening meal. Without carbohydrates, snacking will not put on so much weight as you fear. By this time, you will be able to look a serving of pie à la mode straight in the face without wincing—or pining for it.

2.　*Don't smoke.*　Indirectly, this causes a fall in blood sugar by stimulating the adrenal gland, which in turn influences the liberation of glycogen from the liver.

3.　*Don't drink coffee.*　Its caffeine affects sugar metabolism, causing low blood sugar. It may give you a temporary lift, but you will feel worse after it and become a chain drinker.

4.　*Don't take cola drinks.*　They also contain caffeine in addition to sugar.

Sometimes anxiety and nervousness indirectly cause liberation of too much insulin and produce low blood sugar. Tranquilizers, prescribed by your doctor, are often quite helpful until the diet takes full effect.

Finding the Right Doctor

Purposely, in these few pages I have given you some basic facts about hypoglycemia. Later on, I shall put more flesh on the framework of hypoglycemia.

At this time, I'd like you to be able to ask yourself (and answer), "Am I a wanderer? Have I been riding the medical merry-go-round?"

If so, why? Is it because you are a restless patient and want results right away? Or is it because you do not believe that your doctors have been sufficiently interested and sympathetic to your myriad complaints?

If lack of interest and sympathy is the reason, then you have sufficient motivation for your search for help. Any doctor who tells his patient that his symptoms are all in his head deserves dismissal. He might have been excused before 1924, when Dr. Seale Harris first described the syndrome now known as hypoglycemia, or low blood sugar. But with all the medical publicity about the condition during the intervening years, any modern physician who still refuses to recognize this medical entity is either stubborn or completely deaf and blind to its potential for bringing misery to people.

A few weeks ago an internist of good standing said to me, "I think that this low blood sugar syndrome is being overdone. It's not as important as many doctors believe. Personally, I don't put my nervous patients through six hours of blood sugar tests. I think they are a waste of time."

If that's the kind of doctor you have, then I can understand your becoming a wanderer until you have found one who "believes" when you tell him how badly you feel. As much as I am against patients' jumping on the merry-go-round, I'd be the first to advise you to go looking for the brass ring.

I'd prefer that you do that rather than make your own diagnosis or treat yourself. It is important, if hypoglycemia is present, to determine whether it is organic low blood sugar caused by a defective liver, a tumor in the pancreas, or an inefficient gland such as the adrenal or pituitary. Only your doctor can make the distinction between organic hypoglycemia or idiopathic low blood sugar (cause unknown).

Don't accept the label "neurotic" until you definitely know the status of your blood sugar; until you know whether or not you are suffering from hyperventilation or from low thyroid activity or from some other organic disease. In other words, stop guessing and wondering. You have a right to be a medical shopper, but it's important to know when to call a halt. Indecision is the enemy of the shopper. Once you have found a physician who realizes the importance of hypoglycemia, then drop anchor. Hope that with him to guide you, you will have found your safe harbor.

Where Do You Fit In?

If you are a tired housewife, lacking the strength to climb into bed at night and to get up in the morning, then you need an understanding doctor. If you are in business and continue to complain of exhaustion totally out of proportion to the work you do, then don't accept it as due only to a lazy thyroid gland; make certain that hypoglycemia doesn't play an important part in your enervation.

If you blame your aches and pains and discomforts on

arthritis, ulcer, alcoholism, epilepsy, brain deterioration, change of life, and scores of other reasons—and you don't improve under treatment—consider that your nervousness, fatigue, and other perplexing symptoms may be due to unrecognized low blood sugar. Your blood may have been chronically starved for energy-giving sugar.

Wouldn't it be wonderful to look forward to feeling better? No more irritability or anxiety. No fear of crowds. No fear of being alone. No need for willpower to sit in a theater or ride the subway. No need for grim determination to go to the supermarket. No more insomnia. No more fear of fear.

Impossible? Not at all. Often probable. As you read on, you will realize these are not empty promises. As of now, you can only accept what I say on faith. But later you will get closer to knowing what I know. That will give you confidence, because hypoglycemia will become less a mystery.

2

The Central Station—
Your Pancreas

To overcome your symptoms effectively, you should learn a little about the anatomy and physiology of the pancreas: what happens to cause diabetes, the opposite of low blood sugar; what happens and why during hypoglycemia; why an apparently normal pancreas can cause trouble and be easily overlooked; how too much insulin burns up too much sugar in the blood; how and why you can expect almost miraculous improvement after early recognition and proper treatment of hypoglycemia.

It's only fair to say at this time that I can hardly even begin to describe the complicated workings of the remarkable sugar metabolism of the body. If you are interested in complete details, you can ferret out the information (pictures and diagrams included) about the actual anatomy and physiology of this remarkable organ complex. However, since

19

the purpose of this book is only to make you aware of the clinical aspects of hypoglycemia as they may relate to you personally, I have excluded facts that are necessary only to a medical student.

Anatomy and Physiology

What is important is that you have some idea of how abnormal blood sugar metabolism causes the disagreeable symptoms you complain about. I'll discuss them in a general way, so that you will know why you feel badly; then you can try to be a knowledgeable partner for your doctor, who is trying to help you.

You might call the pancreas a Gemini gland, an organ of two faces. Simultaneously, it performs two important functions: first, it is a ductless endocrine gland that releases the hormone *insulin* into the circulating blood stream to control sugar metabolism in the body (see Figure C); second, it aids in digestion of food by carrying its pancreatic juices through two ducts into the intestine, where it works on breaking down proteins, fats, and carbohydrates. The pancreas itself is a collection of grapelike clusters of glands, about six to eight inches long. The head of the pancreas rests in the curve of the first part of the intestine, which is called the *duodenum.* Its tail extends toward the left. The *islets of Langerhans,* groups of slightly granular cells which secrete the insulin, are most numerous in the tail, although they are scattered throughout the pancreas.

Figure C: Sugar Digestion

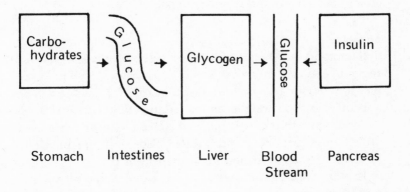

SUGAR TAKEN INTO BODY AS CARBOHYDRATES IS BROKEN DOWN INTO GLUCOSE IN DIGESTIVE TRACT AND STORED IN LIVER AS GLYCOGEN' WHEN BODY NEEDS SUGAR, IT IS REPROCESSED INTO GLUCOSE BEFORE IT ENTERS THE BLOOD STREAM, WHERE IT IS ACTED ON BY INSULIN FROM THE PANCREAS.

When the pancreatic digestive juices fail in their function, the patient gets indigestion (an all-encompassing term that describes any and all kinds of stomach and intestinal discomforts). When the pancreas fails in its important function of controling sugar metabolism, one of two things may happen. If it undersecretes insulin, it may contribute to the onset of diabetes mellitus. If it oversecretes, it may burn up too much blood sugar and produce hypoglycemia.

Diabetes

Symptoms in the unmistakable cases of diabetes are so suggestive that the disease rarely is overlooked. For example, any doctor will become suspicious if you have increased appetite, loss of weight and strength, frequent urination, and excessive thirst. Unexplained itching skin or persistence of leg sores and cuts and bruises also alert the physician to investigate the possibility that diabetes is present.

In the two million who suffer from diabetes without early detection, no outstanding symptoms may be present. Yet the unsuspected disease stealthily inflicts its deleterious effects—causing potential artery degeneration, liability to heart attacks, slow weakening of the kidneys, possible blindness, and other defects.

The reason that early detection is the proper answer to the problem is obvious. Modern early treatment with insulin and diet will allow the diabetic as good a chance as his normal nextdoor neighbor to live out his Biblical quota of years.

Diabetes is hereditary. That should be a tip on whether or not you ought to be especially cautious and go in early for urine and blood examinations. The odds are 100 percent that you may become a diabetic if both of your parents and all of your brothers and sisters are diabetics. The odds are 85 percent if one of your parents, a grandparent, and an aunt or uncle have had it, and about 20 to 25 percent if one of your parents is diabetic. As you can see, the warning often is sufficient — the trick is to take advantage of it.

Hypoglycemia

But don't forget that it is important to obtain blood sugar curves in patients who are just the opposite of diabetics — in those who suffer from abnormally low blood sugar, hyperinsulinism (too much insulin). These people often complain of such vague symptoms as nervousness and fatigue, or of more disabling ones such as tremors, convulsions, and actual coma or unconsciousness.

In my experience, too many people have been labeled neurotics when the real cause is a blood sugar that is either too high or too low.

Sugar Deficiency and Nervousness

Your brain does not have the ability to form and store glycogen (a form of sugar) for future consumption as does the liver. For this reason, the neurons, or brain cells, are dependent from moment to moment on the immediate supply of glucose in the blood. Since oxygen consumption by the brain's cells is tied in with glucose availability, you can see how severe hypoglycemia lowers the oxygen consumption of the brain.

If the loss of sugar is acute, the brain cells can be reinvigorated immediately by taking sugar in some form. The nervousness, irritability, shakes, faintness, and other symptoms disappear. If there is a chronic loss of sugar, though, it is inevitable that some brain cells become so vulnerable that they degenerate and can't be revived. It is evident why sugar deprivation in the brain over a long period of time causes all the disabling symptoms associated with hypoglycemia.

But nature provides backstop protection. Otherwise, every case of hypoglycemia would be mortally serious. When there is an abnormal fall in blood sugar, for one reason or another, a protective system functions through a combination of the nerve-endocrine system of the anterior pituitary gland, the adrenal medulla, and the response of the cells in the pancreas. These three work by blocking the action of insulin secretion by the pancreas, and they stimulate glycogen (sugar reserve) breakdown in the liver, thereby attempting to restore blood sugar to its normal levels.

If these reserve forces are unsuccessful, however, the blood sugar level continues to decline, and the patient suffers anxiety, sweating, rapid pulse, weakness, and trembling of the hands. As the process deepens and the brain cells still are deprived of sugar, the symptoms intensify to disorientation, coarse tremors, and confusion, sometimes followed by convulsions. If the problem is not treated adequately at this time, complications may lead to unconsciousness and death. But if it is recognized early so that the patient may be given sugar solution intravenously (if urgent) or by mouth, all symptoms usually clear up.

Patients with frequent, sudden falls in blood sugar deserve complete study. Are these drops due to tumors of the islet glands of the pancreas? If so, surgery can remove the source of insulin oversecretion and cure the patient. If some other reason is the cause, recovery is not so dramatic.

3

Chronic Fatigue

ONE patient says, "I feel a little tired," and another says, "I feel pooped." There is a wide range between slight tiredness and complete exhaustion. But whichever it is, if it persists for weeks it is the doctor's job to try to find the cause.

Many people think that the most common symptoms are pain, cough, indigestion, headache, and nervousness. Few say fatigue. Yet I believe most doctors will agree that not a day goes by without some patients complaining of this symptom.

Here is a typical example. "I can't understand it. I don't feel sick, but I've been so tired lately; I'm even too exhausted to sit down and eat. Although I haven't been working any harder, I've been exhausted at the end of the day. Comes three o'clock and I have to use all my willpower not to leave my desk and go home to bed. Is this natural? I'm only forty-four years old and haven't any other type of physical discomfort."

Anyone suffering from this extreme degree of fatigue deserves medical investigation. In addition to a complete physical examination, a complete history will be necessary. For example, had he been smoking or drinking too much? How did he sleep—and how long? When did he last have a vacation? Is he bored? Is inner tension due to job hatred causing his tiredness? Does he get enough to eat? Can he relax at home, or is it filled with tension, too?

Suppose the answers to all these questions are negative. Nothing in the patient's way of life indicates the reason for fatigue. Then the doctor must look for organic causes. How is the blood? Any anemia? Fatigue is often a prominent symptom (and sometimes the first) in such conditions as tuberculosis, heart disease, cancer, myasthenia gravis, and scores of other serious diseases.

Now the doctor looks further into this patient's file. His case history indicates that he inadvertently left out some clues. He eats enough, he said, but he has a habit of going without breakfast and taking only two cups of black coffee for lunch. All of his daily caloric intake is concentrated in a large dinner at night.

He admits to other symptoms. He describes what he calls the "shakes or trembles." He actually feels faint in the afternoon. He cannot understand this nervousness: "I have nothing to be nervous about."

Well, the picture is becoming clear. The detective doctor is on a fresh trail. A blood sugar tolerance test ends the chase. There it is on the curve—a definite case of hypoglycemia. In this patient all that is necessary to reduce fatigue and at last remove it entirely is a rearrangement of his diet habits.

An ordinary breakfast, an ordinary light lunch and dinner. In midmorning and midafternoon, a glass of skim milk or a few nuts. Case closed. You might call it the "Case of the Empty Fuel Tank."

Doctor's Dilemma

The management of fatigue is not simple. The doctor is torn between putting the patient through innumerable tests and examinations and trying to save the patient unnecessary expense and loss of time. Fatigue produces other symptoms that mimic many diseases. Therefore, the doctor must choose between making diagnostic shortcuts and putting the patient through the diagnostic mill which includes thorough physical examination, complete history taking, and various laboratory tests and diagnostic maneuvers.

Shall he spare his patient? Or shall he prescribe the works? Often there is the temptation to refer the patient to the psychiatrist early if the symptoms are not clear-cut: the patient has a "low grade infection of undetermined origin," "a borderline thyroid condition," "suffers from overwork and tension." These reasons do not seem sufficient to cause the patient's "nervous exhaustion," so the consultant is called in.

One such patient suffered from anxiety reaction, which she described as deadening fatigue, tremor, excessive sweating, difficulty in falling asleep, weight gain, palpitations, early awakening, phobias, and actual hallucinations. Is it any wonder that her doctor felt helpless in offering a solution to her problem and called for a psychiatrist? But this patient went to three psychiatrists, one psychologist, and several other physicians without finding relief. At last one suggested that her symptoms might fit into the classical syndrome of hypoglycemia. She improved on dietary management, but she still had one complaint.

"Why aren't all doctors aware of this terrible condition? Think of the thousands of people who suffer as I did and don't realize that a simple remedy is right around the corner?"

Finding the Causes

A simple remedy, yes—but not always a simple diagnosis to make. The expert physician must always remember to make sure that fatigue is not really due to just poor living habits or to some organic, underlying illness that is unsuspected. Although hypoglycemia may be a contributing factor, there may be other reasons for day-to-day exhaustion. Short-cuts in diagnosis may not be sufficient to establish the correct one.

Recently, after a meeting, a stranger (call him Mr. Brown) asked me for a curbstone diagnosis. "Doctor, something is sapping my energy. I know it can't be because I'm sick. But I'm always exhausted lately. Any explanation?"

I told Mr. Brown that he was an X quantity and that it was impossible to give him an answer based on my limited knowledge of his case.

"All I know about you," I said, "is that you are a male. I have no idea of your age, occupation, or life style. I don't know whether or not you have recently had a complete physical, or if you're just guessing when you say, 'it can't be that I'm sick.' You must know, I'm sure, that incessant, daily recurring fatigue may be a part of serious illness, too.

"Are you just guessing that you're healthy? Let's assume that you are certain that you do not suffer from heart disease, hypertension, diabetes, cancer, tuberculosis, or some major (or minor) maladies. It's still possible that you may be overlooking more evident reasons for fatigue that can be eliminated without the ministrations of a physician. Perhaps a simple change in way of life is the only essential for feeling better."

I told him to consider the following as possible causes of his exhaustion.

Lack of sleep.   After a nightly deficit, week after week, this lack can add up to chronic fatigue, listlessness, and loss of energy.

Overwork.   Forget that old, frayed aphorism that "work can't hurt anybody." It can if you overdo it. Especially if you are a moonlighter: Working at two jobs lessens the necessary hours for relaxation.

Undervacationing.   The excuse, "I'm too busy to get away," will eventually take its toll in sapping one's energy. Vacationing at regular intervals is not a luxury but a necessity.

Smoking.   Need I add anything to what you have been reading about for years (and seeing on television)? Tobacco will take its toll on your heart, blood vessels, and lungs.

Tension.   Whether at work or at home (or both), it's inevitable that living in tension will deplete your energy perhaps sooner than any other harmful habit. Most people who are otherwise healthy are exhausted because their nerves have been worn to the proverbial frazzle.

Improper diet.   Eating too much will cause obesity, which will tire you. Eating too little will deprive you of the necessary proteins, fats, carbohydrates, minerals, and vitamins. Result? Fatigue.

"I hope you see," I told Mr. Brown, "that all you need to restore your energy is a change in some of your habits. Perhaps the answer is a new way of life. If not, a visit to your doctor certainly is in order.

"Last, but not least, be sure your doctor checks your blood sugar tolerance curve. Fatigue may be due to sugar starvation. You cannot work without fatigue unless the blood sugar level is high enough to furnish the carbohydrates urgently needed by brain cells, muscles, and nerves."

Anyone who is run-down should find out the cause. It may be that all you need is a vacation. But remember that the underlying reason may be low blood sugar. Taking vitamin shots without knowing the real cause of fatigue is like shooting at a target in the dark.

A woman whose job is to raise a family may suffer extreme fatigue. She and others like her should ask themselves these important questions: Do you shop too much, too often, and for too long? Do you clean house with a compulsion to destroy every particle of dust? Do you run your house in helter-skelter fashion, or do you plan your time and try not to cram thirty hours of work into a twenty-four hour day? Do you get sufficient sleep? Do you take time off for an afternoon nap? Have you taken on too many outside obligations, such as bridge club meetings and community organizations?

Take inventory. If self-survey doesn't come up with the answer, then it is time to consult your doctor. Persistent fatigue, as I have mentioned, may be the first warning of illness. Whether the trouble is organic or emotional, proper treatment may provide you with a reservoir of new energy.

However, if you are still tired something important may have been overlooked—your blood sugar. If your doctor hasn't taken it for one reason or another, you have the right to suggest a blood sugar tolerance test. If he's still adamant and is sure (without the ·test) that your blood sugar level is not a factor, then you have the right to ask for consultation—or change doctors.

The Need for Rest

Most of us "wouldn't be caught dead in a hammock." We rebel at the "lazy" label. We don't like to be called soft.

Nevertheless, the efficient machine is the periodically rested machine. You can run a high powered car for hundreds of miles at high speeds and it will not fall apart suddenly, like the "one-hoss shay." But keep up that pace, day after day, and the glistening chrome and smooth-acting engine will be ready for the junk heap. It will deteriorate many thousands of miles earlier than its sister car that has had a modicum of care.

Human machines are similar. Remember that people operate on different levels of efficiency. Some are like the latest model Cadillac, Lincoln, or Imperial. Others are born with a body model equivalent to a five-year-old jalopy that has already become a member of the 100,000-mile club.

You have undoubtedly heard some people say, "I was born tired." They get along all right when they don't race their own motors because they think they are as durable as the next fellow. It's better to know your engine and run it according to its horsepower. You will go farther, even if not so fast.

I once saw a forty-one-year-old executive of a large corporation. His complaint was tiredness to the point of exhaustion. This man had an expensive make of body machine. Nature has been kind to him. He was 6 feet 1 inch tall; he weighed 190 pounds.

What about this man? Why did he suffer from chronic exhaustion? He wasn't the type who was "born tired." As he told it, "Doctor, I guess I've just been burning out my motor. You see before you a fool."

I asked him to elaborate.

"I'm my own worst enemy. I've been giving myself a terrible beating for years. I'm not the kind of fellow who can sit down for a half-hour and relax. I can't read a book, finish a newspaper, or just sit and chat for hours. Call me 'fidgety Phil.'"

He looked at me sheepishly and continued, "All my life I've been driven to be on the go. I went in for athletics at school. I've given business the same college try. No vacations, twelve hours of work every day—and taking it home with me at night. At the office, if the elevator is slow in getting to me I think nothing of climbing three flights of stairs, taking two or three steps at a time. You see before you a human dynamo that's just about run down. I only hope there's enough of it left for you to do a rewinding job."

I have seen all kinds of go-getters. Many of them won't admit they're wrong. They have lost all perspective. They are like the compulsively driven ant or bee. But this man admitted his indiscretions; so there was hope for him. Fortunately, he was still organically well. What he needed was good advice to keep his machine from falling apart. In effect, here is what I told him.

"Plan to take off a few weeks right now. You have forty-eight hours in which to make arrangements and pack. While you are away, you are to be in bed ten hours every night. You are to nap for an hour every afternoon. You may play nine holes of golf a day, no more. No tennis. No overly long walks. Swim a little, read a little, play cards in moderation—but relax a lot.

"During your vacation, you will have time to ask, and perhaps answer, these questions: What's the rush? Where am I going? From where does this work compulsion come? Am I running away from my wife? from my children? Am I insecure? Has the almighty dollar or position in the community blinded me to the really important things in life?"

He grinned. "That seems like easy advice to take. Anything else?"

I answered that the most difficult part would be the readjustment to a sane way of life when he returned. "Resolve to work no more than eight hours a day. Take at least one-and-a-half hours for lunch, outside your office. Your desk top should be cleared for working, not for eating. Besides, warm milk and a stale cheese sandwich are for a mouse— not for a man.

"Resolve to break up your working day by frequent short periods of relaxation. For example, a fifteen-minute nap on a couch. A sprawl in your chair with feet atop your desk. Refuse to answer the telephone during these vacuum periods.

"Resolve, for a while, to get into bed by nine o'clock two or three nights a week. And remember, all this will take a lot of practice. It won't come easy. But it will be worth it when you consider that it will lick your fatigue."

As he left, I wished him good luck—and crossed my fingers. (He died two years later of a coronary attack. He refused to, or couldn't slow his motor. Couldn't find a new way of life.)

The human body is not the answer to perpetual motion. It will seemingly go on endlessly, without complaint, and then suddenly bog down. I have seen many such break- downs in men who held down two jobs, thinking they could work eighteen hours a day indefinitely.

I know businessmen who brag about working twelve to sixteen hours a day. Ask one when he had his last vacation and he will smile and say, "Don't remember ever having one. Not in the last fifteen years, anyway." These men do not re- alize they are greasing their own toboggans for a ride to oblivion.

But not all businessmen commit slow suicide. I asked one man recently to give me his secret formula for his apparent fitness and good health. "You don't take vacations," I said. "Yet you seem fit and rested. Just how do you do it?"

He was a successful businessman of about fifty. He was relaxed and looked far from tired.

"I learned long ago," he said, "that waiting forty-eight or

fifty weeks for a vacation doesn't make sense. If I did that, I couldn't last out the year. The secret, I think, is short, frequent rest periods. I divide these into daily rests and bimonthly rests.

"I've learned to take a half-hour nap after lunch. I also take one after dinner if we plan to go out in the evening. You'd be surprised how this daily hour of rest revitalizes my engine.

"But I consider the bimonthly rest equally as important. Every two weeks throughout the year, on Friday night, my wife and I hole in at an out-of-town hotel. On Saturday we sleep late and have brunch brought up. A show Saturday night, after-theater dinner, and then back to the hotel. Brunch again on Sunday, and then we're on our way home.

"I tell you, doctor, I wouldn't swap this regime for a yearly six-week or two-month vacation. My own son and daughter-in-law have adopted this short-vacation habit, too. They have discovered that it acts as a pick-me-up for young fathers or mothers who are exhausted by the cares and responsibilities of raising a family.

"Oh, there's one more thing that's important. I'm careful about what I eat. My wife has hypoglycemia. She has learned to stay away from sweets and eat a wholesome diet. I do the same. I've never had a blood sugar taken myself. But I eat often and well anyway. I guess watching my diet and taking frequent vacations are the reasons I never know what it means to be tired like so many of my friends."

Other Causes of Fatigue

If fatigue persists in spite of proper daily living habits or a remedial diet in hypoglycemia, another look and frequent reviews in the diagnostic procedure are necessary. Questions must be asked and answered by further tests. For example, here are some organic conditions in which the early effects may be continuing fatigue and exhaustion of undetermined origin—and which are discovered only by special examinations:

Diabetes mellitus   (the opposite of hypoglycemia)

Anemia   (important to determine whether or not it is secondary anemia due to iron deficiency or bleeding, or is pernicious anemia or some other primary anemia)

Arthritis   (of all types)

Polycythemia   (too many red blood cells, sometimes cause unknown, at other times due to heart or lung disease)

Hyperthyroidism   (overactive thyroid)

Hypothyroidism   (underactive, or lazy, thyroid)

Pus in urine   (may be due to chronic bladder or kidney infection, or to cystitis due to stone or tumor in the bladder or kidneys)

Adrenal insufficiency   (as in Addison's disease)

Malnutrition   (due to inadequate diet and vitamin deficiencies)

Leukemia   (in which there is a disturbance in white blood cells)

Acute and chronic infections   (such as tuberculosis, hepatitis, or brucellosis)

Diseases of the nervous system (such as Parkinson's disease, narcolepsy, small strokes, myasthenia gravis)

Heart diseases

Cancer

This is only a partial list of often overlooked causes of fatigue. It is important for you to know this small core of varying conditions so that you will not fall into the trap of believing that hypoglycemia management is the cure-all for fatigue and many other symptoms I have enumerated.

Each patient deserves personalized investigation and thorough study. But this includes blood sugar study, too. As I have been saying, it is too often overlooked in the search for the more serious conditions I have enumerated. It is lost in the maze of diagnostic tests for other diseases.

4

Narcolepsy

I F you suffer from insomnia, you know how distressing and fearsome it is to get into bed night after night and actually fight for the welcome forgetfulness of a deep sleep. To thrash around all night in wakefulness, wondering how you will ever get through another working day, can soon become the reason for chronic, debilitating fatigue and frustration. Millions of insomniacs will attest to this.

But there is the opposite side of the coin, the inability to stay awake. Although not so common as insomnia, narcolepsy is also hard to bear. Here is one patient's experience.

"I have had a difficult job staying awake since I was about 20 years old. One day I'm going to kill myself and some innocent people. Not because I want to but because I can't stay awake at the wheel of my car. Years ago, while driving, I awoke to find the front of my car under a tractor

37

trailer. How we all got out of it alive and without serious injuries I'll never know.

"Quite often, later, I'd fall asleep behind the wheel. At first I thought it was a form of road hypnosis, until I realized it often happened when I was cruising slowly on the city streets. I am now twenty-eight, have everything to live for—three kids, a new home, a wonderful wife—but I have been fighting for my life behind the wheel of a car for the past eight years.

"Every day going home (ten miles away) I start falling asleep after the first two miles. Many times I miss the turns I want. Even after I pull over and take a half-hour nap, I still have to fight the urge to sleep at least fifteen times before I reach home. I feel very lucky to get there.

"I seem to be in a twilight zone. I fall asleep while making out my worksheet. I am a printing pressman and I have fallen asleep standing next to the press. I catch myself as my knees buckle just before hitting the floor. If I sit down to work, I fall asleep in five minutes.

"Even if I'm occupied without distractions, I cannot stay awake for any length of time; even after six to ten hours of sleep. I have fallen asleep with smelling salts in my hand while driving. I could give thousands of similar examples.

" I asked a doctor about my condition, and all he did was prescribe smelling salts and say I might need to see a psychiatrist later."

This patient's dietary history was an interesting one. Like many others, he believed in what I call the dog diet, one large meal at night. He would leave home without even a hot drink in the morning. While others at the shop went out for lunch, he would nap. When he came home at night, he would "eat a meal big enough for three." Then he would dip into the refrigerator all evening whenever commercials disturbed his television watching. He was at least fifty pounds overweight. On prodding, he recalled that he always had "faintness and nervous feelings" during the day.

His history was certainly suggestive of narcolepsy. After discovering hypoglycemia, I suggested a turnabout in diet regime before putting him on any medication: a large breakfast, a medium-sized lunch, and a dinner without second helpings. I also prescribed snacks in midmorning, midafternoon and before he went to bed—basically, a low carbohydrate diet.

Within two weeks, his drowsiness was at least 75 percent improved. After taking Ritalin to help overcome his unnatural sleepiness, he said that for the first time in years he felt like a normal human being again. His horrendous nightmare days had been transformed into serene and livable ones.

Three Causes in Traffic Accidents

Think of auto accidents and you think of alcohol. And for good reason. Approximately 50 percent of the deaths on our highways and streets are in some way related to alcohol in the drivers—and often in the pedestrians involved.

But, as you can see, alcohol isn't the only threat. Many drugs, overlooked and underestimated, can cause accidents too. Of course, it is evident that LSD, marijuana, amphetamine and heroin users are unstable and dangerous drivers. Nevertheless, millions of people who take tranquilizers, sedatives, and antihistamines may not be aware that potential danger is around the corner when they also drive.

It is inevitable that drugs that act on your brain will slow your reflexes, sometimes to the point of making you drowsy and actually causing you to fall asleep as you drive. So before you drive, review your medicine intake. When did you take it last? Has it worn off sufficiently so that you are alert enough to guide your machine through traffic?

The sleepy driver obviously equals (or exceeds) the intoxicated driver in threatening his own life and the lives of others. You are constantly warned not to drink before driving; certainly you should be warned not to drive when sleepy. Another overlooked cause of highway accidents is drivers who suffer from narcolepsy. In a recent study, about 80 percent of patients with narcolepsy reported driving while drowsy; 40 percent of these patients actually fell asleep while driving.

Narcolepsy and Hypoglycemia

"I have a problem that is beginning to interfere with every phase of my life. I am a compulsive eater. Within the past six months, my life has turned into a nightmare. Every day I eat to the point of becoming physically ill. I'm becoming quite fat. And what's worse, I'm always sleepy lately. No matter how much rest I get at night, I am sure to be fighting to stay awake.

"I feel that I am perhaps using food as an alcoholic uses liquor. Willpower alone doesn't seem to be the answer. I feel there must be a deeper reason for such gorging. I don't know where to turn because I am really ashamed of myself. I have not revealed my weakness to anyone, haven't even told my husband.

"I can't imagine the reason for this terrible habit. I am a very happily married twenty-four-year-old with a wonderful husband who has the promise of a bright future. There seemingly is no reason for my self-indulgence. Please, please help me if you can. I am desperate."

Nervous and always sleepy. Whenever I encounter this combination of complaints in a patient, I am not satisfied until I order a six-hour glucose tolerance test. I told this woman that I could not come up with a magic formula to turn off her insatiable desire for food until she herself found a strong motivation to lose weight.

"Trying to save a wonderful marriage is motivation enough," I said. "Why not think of what your excess weight and continual sleepiness will do to your marriage? I think that after a while you will be strong enough to prevent your hand from reaching our for food."

I suggested that she cut out most carbohydrates and go on a high protein diet. No more box-of-candy shindigs; no more ice cream sodas or banana splits; no more loading up on half-a-dozen or more slices of bread at every meal.

"In addition to narcolepsy," I told her, "your blood sugar curve indicates that you have hypoglycemia. Helping one will help the other. Spread your meals over six to eight stops for food. Small helpings, low in carbohydrates, and no full-course dinners at night. I'll write you a prescription for Ritalin that will help keep you awake."

Within weeks came the expected transformation. New dresses, new suits, new outlook on life; a trim, wide-awake wife for a happier husband to come home to. No longer did he call her sleepyhead.

If you have a similar problem—always sleepy, always hungry—don't hesitate to take it up with your physician. Why be ashamed to confess that you overeat and are "lazy all the time"? Often only your doctor can discover the reason for your unnatural craving for food and difficulty in keeping awake.

Becoming Aware of Narcolepsy

In my own practice, I have seen many innocent hypogly-cemia patients who were sleeping their lives away. Sometimes they had been accused of boredom, of being lazy good-for-nothings, of being unambitious. Even the medical profession's increased awareness has not prevented many overlooked cases. They have been misdiagnosed as borderline hypothyroids or as a slight anemias. Yet when thyroid extract or iron or other medication didn't help, the diagnosis still remained a question mark. A blood sugar tolerance test might easily have solved the problem and converted them into energetic and much happier people.

The term "narcolepsy"-comes from a combination of the Greek words *narke,* meaning stupor, and *lepsis,* meaning seizure. In most cases of narcolepsy, which affects about 0.3 percent of the population, the true origin has not been recognized. Thus, over a half-million Americans wear such false labels as sleepyhead, stupid, lazy, because their families and friends (and their doctors) are unaware that they do indeed suffer from some medical disability and not from an imaginary illness. Only those who fight and struggle to stay awake during the day realize what it is to suffer and bear (at the same time) the taunts of those closest to them.

For example, a man goes to sleep while playing cards. His partner, waiting for a reply to a bid, looks up, astounded, to see him taking a nap while holding his cards. Again, a young girl falls asleep while eating. Her attack may resemble petit mal of epilepsy but is actually due to narcolepsy complicated by low blood sugar. Many similar cases are helped by a low carbohydrate, high protein diet and administration of Ritalin or similar medication.

In about 75 percent of patients, narcolepsy appears before the age of twenty-five. It may develop during early adolescence or in the second and third decades of life. It is more common in the male. I have had quite a few patients who were formerly athletes of note, big fellows who had allowed themselves to become too fat.

In some patients with narcolepsy, these sleepy feelings come on as many as a dozen or more times a day. Some immediately will be rendered "slow and stupid" after a heavy noon meal. The rest of the day is a battle to stay awake and work. Others fall asleep at concerts or at the theater. These "naps" last anywhere from a few seconds to fifteen minutes. Although refreshment should result from these interludes, they often cause depression and tiredness.

Close questioning of the patient often will result in a diagnosis that may otherwise be overlooked. For example, the person may say, "About once a day or every other day I get an attack of weakness in my legs and suddenly sink to the ground. I'm aware of my surroundings but feel as if I've had a bad dream. I can't move, but I know everything that is going on. It lasts only a minute or so, but it's awfully embarrassing and disturbing."

This condition, which appears in about two out of three patients with narcolepsy, is called cataplexy—a sudden decrease in muscle tone. And about one of every three cases of narcolepsy has what are called "hypnagogic hallucinations."

If the diagnosis of narcolepsy is still unsure, then brain wave examination will help. You also may be given a drug test, using Ritalin, Benzedrine, Desoxyn, or Dexedrine.

But even with drug therapy, diet should not be forgotten. No patient will find real improvement if his hypoglycemia is overlooked and untreated.

Narcolepsy can be worse than insomnia. "Oh, for a good day's wakefulness" is often more important than "Oh, for a good night's sleep."

Thousands of miserable people drag themselves through life with superhuman effort to stay alive, even though they function much below the levels of their potential capacities. Youngsters in grade school are called stupid; high school students barely make it through to graduation; questing but inordinately sleepy young people fail to negotiate college or the responsibilities of business. They hope that as adults they will grow out of their deficiencies and drawbacks—that somehow a good fairy or mother nature will instill them with energy so that they can graduate, or save their jobs, or have normal social lives, or save their marriages.

But too many fail for one simple reason. They have been tagged with a label they do not deserve to wear. They are not lazy. They are not sleepy because they are ambitionless. They are not stupid. They are not idiots. They continue to suffer simply because a diagnosis has been overlooked.

Although narcolepsy and hypoglycemia are not invariably associated, you will need more than willpower to transform you into a normal social being if you overlook the possibility that they may occur together. Some of the responsibility is yours. If you hope to improve, insist on study of your blood sugar tolerance. Insist on electroencephalograms if necessary. Do something, do anything—except willingly go along living as you have. Too many resign themselves because they believe, "I've been born this way. There's nothing I can do to help myself." More often than you realize, you are the master of your fate.

5

Change in Personality

Brain cells need sugar to burn just as they need an oxygen supply to burn it. To function normally, we require sugar now, not later. Otherwise, we suffer the common symptoms of sugar deprivation that I have mentioned.

We know that sudden, acute sugar loss can be replaced and symptoms cleared up in a jiffy. But chronic sugar loss at last affects sensitive brain cells. The result may be an actual change in personality.

Some Simple Experiments

Here are some simple tests to determine how low blood sugar produces change in personality. Observe yourself or, better still, observe your children. The child who has been out running and playing and wrestling with other kids all afternoon often comes into the house grouchy and testy.

45

Within minutes after he eats dinner he becomes a little angel—quiet and tractable and pleasant. If you had given the child a couple of peanut butter sandwiches in midafternoon, you might have prevented the later irritability.

Your spouse? A fine, even-tempered person? Easy to get along with? How does this mate act after a long day's work? Especially on days when "I didn't even have time for a sandwich." Lack of food may temporarily turn an even-tempered person into an ill-tempered monster.

How about you? If you have been busy, you may not have taken the time for a midafternoon snack. Some actually reasonable request may cause you to snap for no good reason. You realize, suddenly, that you are hungry. You take a glass of milk or bit of cheese, and within minutes you are sorry for having spoken so harshly. You have become a philosopher.

Personality changes? True. Temporary, yes. But probably all dependent on a low blood sugar that has turned the brain into an irritable piece of living machinery.

Some Examples

The three cases that follow differ in their symptoms, but in all three the cause is the same—hypoglycemia.

Fear

"I was a happy-go-lucky woman until my twenties when I had a complete change in personality. I became scared and anxious. It all began after I had a miscarriage and came close to bleeding to death. At the hospital they did a D and C, and I came out of it all right.

"However, after I got home I found I got frightened around lunchtime every day. I became frightened because I felt as if I were going to faint. I thought maybe I had claustrophobia; so I took my young daughter out in the backyard where we sat and ate lunch in the sunshine and fresh air. Although I was shaking when I was out there, I felt all right again when I came back in.

"My husband was building a large addition to our house, but after three months of being scared to death, I asked him one Saturday to stay in the house with me because I was frightened. I was afraid of fainting. When I told him about it, he marched me off to the doctor because he felt he couldn't take any time off from his work.

"I had not gone to our doctor because a visit was quite costly, and we were putting all our money into the building of our house. We also had to help in supporting my husband's parents and my mother in addition to our expenses in bringing up our own three children.

"The doctor said that if I didn't get over my silly fears pretty soon I'd have to go to a psychiatrist. He said that my fear of fainting was a delayed reaction to my narrow brush with death during the hemorrhage that followed my miscarriage. I was so embarrassed that I started to cry. Then I began to laugh. Go to a psychiatrist? We hardly could stand the expense of seeing our family doctor.

"After we left the doctor's office, I realized that I couldn't depend on his medical advice. Anyone who suggested a psychiatrist after only one visit, without taking any special tests to see what was really wrong with me, was someone I couldn't have any confidence in.

"I decided I'd have to depend on myself. So I read up on anxiety. I came across an article that discussed low blood sugar. I recognized myself in a case history I read there. This woman also feared that she'd faint when left alone. She felt trembly and nervous as I did. But she got well after she discovered that she had hypoglycemia.

"So I decided to stake some small savings on a visit to another doctor, who agreed to send me to a laboratory for a blood sugar tolerance test. Sure enough, they found a low blood sugar curve. My new doctor put me on a high protein, low carbohydrate diet. During the acute spells, before the diet took hold, I'd dump a tablespoonful of sugar into a glassful of water and drink it down.

"It was like raising a curtain that was coming down over my eyes and mind. Immediately I felt all right. Then I began to realize that it wasn't the sunshine and getting out-of-doors that had made me feel better for a little while. It was the lunch!

"After I had been on the special diet only a few weeks, my husband said, 'What a change in personality! You're like the girl I always knew.'

"I felt so well that I mixed mortar and helped my husband lay brick. I learned to saw with a power saw, hammer nails, and buy lumber, besides doing all the housework for my family. I also had the courage to hire carpenters, plumbers, and stone masons when we did not know how to do the work.

"When our house is built, I'm going to call it our Sugar House. My husband agrees that it will be a good name for the house, but he also insists on the nickname 'Sugar' for me. It used to be 'Baby,' but 'Sugar,' the way he says it, sounds just as sweet.

"In spite of it all, it makes me actually sick to think of how many innocent people are suffering from a changed personality because they don't realize that low blood sugar is the cause of their misery."

Daily Headaches

"I've had headaches every day. It's an unnatural way to get fun out of life. I'm only in my mid-thirties, but I act as if I were in my forties or fifties and going through a terrible period of change. My personality seems warped. I notice it. My husband and friends notice it. Our three kids notice it.

I'm not the reasonable, easy-going mother and wife I was only a short while ago. Trying to get relief from patented pain killers has been unsuccessful.

"I've been a perfectly healthy woman except for a vaginal hysterectomy seven years ago and an emergency appendectomy two years before that. I began to get headaches when I was six months pregnant with our oldest son. They didn't bother me much then, but lately they have been so bad and so persistent that I go to bed with them and wake up with them. I've consulted several doctors. Each says that I can't possibly have these daily headaches for such a long period of time. But I live with them. I'm not imagining the pain!

"I know that if I could rid myself of these headaches my health would be perfect. I'd become a reasonable human being again, as easy to live with as I was when we first got married. I have no other complaints, but the headaches get worse as the days go by. The moment I mention my problem to a doctor he takes off on anything but what I'm there for.

"I'm desperate for help. I can stand back and look at myself, and I don't like myself as I am. I want to be *me,* the me I used to be. I'm tired of taking aspirin and tranquilizers, and of being put down by everyone as a hopeless complainer."

With this patient, considerable work was necessary. She agreed to undergo various tests and to see specialists in allergies, the nervous system, the eyes, ears, nose, and throat, as well as her dentist.

Physically, she was all right. Nothing in her home life indicated that husband or children might be contributing to tension headaches. She had no recognizable allergies. Everything came up zero in diagnosis.

Except for one finding. You guessed it. She had a low blood sugar curve. Unquestionably low. Like other patients, she ran true to form when six small meals were substituted for her usual haphazard way of eating. Within months she had regained the twenty pounds she had lost during the previous year. Her nerves quieted down without the aid of tranquilizers. She hadn't uncapped an aspirin bottle in weeks. And her husband made the usual confirmation: "She's a different girl. No, she's the same girl she used to be."

As I mentioned earlier, not every headache, not every ache and pain, not every disagreeable variation from previous sweetness and light can be charged to hypoglycemia. However, as I also said earlier, no examination of a patient can be considered complete unless the glucose tolerance test is part of the investigation, especially in those patients who have been on the medical merry-go-round and are still frustrated in their search for the elusive brass ring.

Bad Temper

"My husband has developed a disagreeable personality that has become worse during the past few months. Although he never was a particularly happy man, he was usually kind, pleasant, and loving toward our children and me. Then he gradually began to change into a completely selfish, dissatisfied, complaining grouch.

"Throughout our married life, although he has not been able to earn a great deal of money, we always had a nice clean house and enough food and clothing. I have worked most of the time and have never complained. I have been perfectly satisfied with our standard of living. Now, suddenly, my husband feels that life is passing him by. He is forty-five. He complains that because of the children and me he cannot do all the things he wants to do in his lifetime. He says that we are the burdens who are keeping him from his great loves—travel and hunting expeditions with his friends—and from possessing the material things that other men have.

"He gets into sullen, self-pitying moods that are usually followed by a temper flare-up. Once he slapped me right in front of the children. He had a complete checkup two years ago when he was out of town, and the doctor found him in good health. I have begged him to have an examination, but he adamantly states that it is I, not his physical condition, that is at fault."

After much prodding and gentle nagging, this man agreed to an examination. He appeared to be quiet and gentle, but you never can judge by outward appearances.

I said, "Your wife has given me permission to repeat what she has told me about your behavior. She says that although she is becoming quite nervous, she is more concerned about your effect on the children. Particularly the youngest cannot understand the change in you. What is your story? There are always two sides."

"I agree," he said. "I've felt a change in my personality. I take everything so seriously these days. I'm easily depressed, and it has been showing up at the office, too. I try to keep myself reined in, but the wild horses get away at times. I lose my temper, and I admit I'm hard to live with. I'm sorry for my wife and kids. I suppose I'm going through the male change—I've read about that. That's probably the reason I'm acting as I do. Like any other married man, or even bachelor, I have my regrets about what I might have done with my life. But it has become, I realize, too exaggerated in importance. I have good reason to be a happy man. Perhaps you can help."

His physical examination was negative, but a routine blood sugar determination disclosed that he was hypoglycemic.

"I can find only two reasons for the way you have been feeling," I said. "I believe that you're going through the male climacteric, commonly called male change of life. But you have abnormally low blood sugar, too. With your history of heavy coffee drinking, large consumption of alcohol 'to steady your nerves,' and a mixed-up diet pattern in which you fill up on sweets of all kinds when you get hunger and fainting sensations during the day, I can't help but believe that low blood sugar is intensifying your symptoms."

He cut his coffee to two cups a day, took only one highball before dinner, and eliminated most sweets ("I used to eat chocolates by the boxful"). He quickly improved at least 50 percent, and within six months, he was, according to his wife, his "old sweet self."

6

Dizziness

Two doctors sat down after a medical meeting to talk shop, as doctors usually do. One of them said, "Bill, what would you say is the most common complaint among your patients over forty?"

Bill thought a while and then said, "I'd guess that it's rheumatism. You know, the aches and pains older patients complain about, whether they have or haven't got bad arthritic changes in their joints. They say they feel stiff when they get up in the morning, and it takes a while for the joints to oil up. Or they complain that it's hard for them to get out of a chair after they've been sitting for a while. Aches and pains in muscles, nerves, and joints certainly seem to be a natural accompaniment of getting on in years. What's been your experience, Frank?"

The second doctor answered, "I agree with what you say,

but here's a symptom that's a close runner-up—dizziness. Don't you find that to be true in your practice?"

Both doctors agreed and went on to discuss other things.

Some Causes

While it is true, for example, that headache is also a common complaint of young and old alike, dizziness seems to have predilection for those over thirty-five or forty. What are its causes? What can be done about it?

In the young, dizziness usually is due to disturbances in the eyes or ears. Many a case of dizziness has been cleared up by proper glasses. Many others respond to treatment of the middle-ear disease we call Ménière's syndrome. Of course, some dizziness in the younger group may be due to anemia or to any acute disease-produced fever complicated by a labrynthitis. It also may be caused by a chronic anxiety state.

But dizziness in the older age groups seems to be tied up mostly with a physiological change in blood circulation. Some persons learn to accept it as they do gray hair or wrinkles. At first, they are thrown emotionally off balance by the realization that the machine is not the smooth performer it used to be a few years back. Then, if philosophical, they accept these motor sputterings as something inevitable in everybody's life.

It is also true that in persons over forty dizziness may be a result of errors in refraction, middle-ear imbalance, and anxiety states. The major cause, though, may lie in the arteries and brain circulation. For example, high blood pressure is a common cause of dizzy spells, but the intensity varies among patients.

Some Treatments

It is evident that daily recurring dizziness deserves investigation. If the diagnosis is high blood pressure, heart disease, or kidney disease, these conditions should be treated by a physician. If the trouble is Ménière's disease, the problem may be a stubborn one. Cutting down on salt intake and taking antivertigo drugs and histamine preparations may limit the intensity of the attacks. If dizziness cannot always be eliminated, it can be lessened. If the cause seems to be old-fashioned hardening of the arteries, then you should learn to live within your limitations, be philosophical, be thankful that you lived long enough to feel this way (which, I admit, is not much help during the actual attack of dizziness).

In the rarest of cases, dizziness that comes on suddenly and seems to get worse as the weeks go by may be due to a brain tumor. If all other causes of dizziness have been ruled out, tumor should be considered, especially if the dizziness is aggravated by sudden change of position and is accompanied by vomiting and severe headache. However, it is reassuring to know that the odds are greatly against dizziness that is caused by tumor.

The cause really may be trivial. Many patients say, "I'm sure to feel dizzy and light-headed if I don't have a bowel movement every day."

To sum up, first look to the common causes of dizziness. Have your eyes refracted; then have your ears checked. If you still haven't found the cause, have a complete physical examination. This will be a double check on your heart, arteries, blood pressure, kidneys, and blood. If your doctor can't find the cause, he may refer you to a neurologist, who will go over your entire nervous system to rule out serious disease.

Suppose the dizziness persists. Are you going to accept it, just as others accept stubborn stiffness in the joints, obstinate ringing in the ears, and hundreds of other discomforts? Dizziness, like any other symptom, requires study to determine its true source. If one coughs, is it due to ordinary viral infection? pneumonia? bronchitis? emphysema? tuberculosis? lung cancer? If one has "pain in the stomach," is the reason too many green apples? Acute gastritis due to too much alcohol? A gall bladder attack? Acute appendicitis? Such symptoms and their causes are innumerable.

I have not yet mentioned one possible cause of dizziness—abnormally low blood sugar. In many who suffer from dizziness, hypoglycemia may be overlooked as the sole or contributing cause.

Three Examples

"I haven't got high blood pressure. I do not have heart disease, and yet I've been awfully bothered by dizziness and loss of balance for the past few weeks. It all seemed to come on after a bad virus attack. At times, I actually stagger around. My doctor says the cure is time. He hasn't prescribed any medication. He says it's likely that my dizziness is due to some spasm in the blood vessels of my brain. But I'm only forty-seven. Isn't that too young for that problem? Is there anything else I can do to help myself? The condition seems to be getting worse."

I told this patient that the causes of dizziness must be sought out carefully and patiently. I agreed that dizziness can be a disturbing and disabling symptom. I referred her to an ear specialist, who found that her trouble was due to labrynthitis—an imbalance in the delicate organs of the inner ear. Often the dizziness leaves without treatment; at other times special attention to various contributing factors is necessary. In her case, I found a low blood sugar curve. It seems that after her virus attack she had changed her dietary habits completely, eating infrequently and indulging in sweets.

After a few weeks on a high protein, low carbohydrates diet combined with between-meal snacks, she lost all of her disquieting dizzy feelings. Of course, as in many cases, time alone might have helped her labrynthitis. However, it is likely that her hypoglycemia was a contributing cause of her discomforts.

"I have been getting dizzy every morning lately. I am eighty years old. At first I blamed it on my age, but I had a doctor who doesn't treat people by how old they are. He took a blood sugar tolerance test, which was low. I had been eating like a fool. No meat, no fish, no eggs. Practically living on coffee, doughnuts, and bread and jam. Since the test and the new diet, I haven't had a dizzy spell. Two earlier doctors told me it was poor circulation in the brain. Bosh!"

Dizziness quite often is associated with a deficient diet. Overweight people who go on crash diets not only complain of weakness but also say, "I've been so dizzy I can't stand."

Youngsters are not immune to freaky diets. Either they will go without breakfast and drink only a soda for lunch, or they will eliminate necessary proteins from their diets because some young friend has told them that they ought to go on a vegetarian diet. When dizziness becomes a problem, both doctor and patient often overlook poor nutrition as a cause.

"Recently I went to another doctor because I had constant dizziness. Sometimes while in bed with my eyes closed I would feel a whirling sensation [vertigo], which disappeared as soon as I opened my eyes. Then I would stand up and get dizzy all over again. Tranquilizers helped only for a while. I am almost back to where I was before.

"I was sent to a neurologist, who took an electro-encephalogram. This EEG was normal. But what worries me is this:

Could a mistake have been made in the interpretation of the EEG? You see, I was very nervous and dizzy that day. When the operator of the machine told me to relax and close my eyes, I had to force them closed. I told him that I was very nervous. I think I shouldn't have told him, because now I think that maybe something abnormal turned out in the EEG, and he thought it was due only to nerves. Is such a mistake possible?

"I still have the dizziness and the vertigo. I am 20 years old, married, and proud of my figure, and I am not taking any birth control pills or any other drugs. I'm concerned that the dizziness is caused by some trouble in my brain. Do you think it's possible that being on a strictly vegetarian diet might be making me sick? My dizziness didn't begin until I went on this diet. It has done wonders for my figure, but I'd rather feel well than look well."

She had made her own diagnosis. The big clue was easy to see. She had hypoglycemia. She went back to a sensible eating routine, and within weeks the dizziness disappeared. And, thankfully, her figure stayed the same because of the low intake of carbohydrates.

A Warning

"I don't drink coffee or tea, and I have never smoked or taken alcohol. I am thirty-five, newly married, and under a doctor's care for anxiety and nervousness. I have no children. I have been on tranquilizers for a few years, especially lately when I have been complaining of dizziness. I had a fasting blood sugar test a few years ago. The doctor said it was 88 and normal, and I did not need any special diet. He told me to suck on some hard candies whenever I got these dizzy spells and felt especially nervous.

"Today I am home because I'm suffering from fatigue.

Last week I played tennis and swam. Right after swimming, I felt dizzy. I felt as if weights were attached to my body, and I started to shake all over.

"What do you think of this incident? The shakes and dizziness happen so often lately that I'm beginning to lose confidence in myself. My husband wants to go out and socialize, but I insist on staying home. You can imagine what this will do to our marriage."

Trembly? Shaky? Dizzy? All point to hypoglycemia. The answer to her problem seems so evident. But hold on. A six-hour blood sugar tolerance curve is normal. She is not a fortunate candidate for early improvement. In her case, all symptoms were part of a chronic anxiety state. She suffered for a few years before psychotherapy, tranquilizers, and a patient husband brought about substantial improvement.

Moral? A case history like this jolts one into the realization that hypoglycemia is not the universal cause of nervousness, and its treatment is not some kind of abracadabra that will open the lock to a life free from all anxiety and its associated symptoms. Certainly, keep looking for it. Always be aware that hypoglycemia may be an offender. But see it in true perspective. Not a cure-all, not a catchall, but a *cure-some*. And the some may run into quite a few thousands of unhappy, anxious people who might be helped by not overlooking the possibility that they could be suffering from hypoglycemia.

7

Headaches and Hypoglycemia

Sometimes without actually trying to eavesdrop, one hears medical case histories on planes or buses. While sitting next to two women on a city bus, I heard one say, "I think my doctor is a doll. He's so interested when you don't feel well. Even a headache is reason enough for him to be compassionate and not just say, 'Take a couple of aspirin.'

"One day I came to his office complaining of having these terrible headaches. I told him I was nervous and shaky most of the day, too. Know what he said? 'Better take a glucose tolerance test. I want to make sure your blood sugar is OK.'

"Well, I took it. And guess what? I really do have low blood sugar. I've been on my diet pretty faithfully for about three months now. The shakes are gone, and the headaches come on only for an hour or so when I try to do too much.

"What a relief! When I think of how I used to wake up with headaches and go to sleep with them. I used to feel light-headed and get so nervous I'd feel like screaming. If my doctor weren't the suspicious type, I'm sure I'd have gone from one doctor to another for years, and no one would have found out that I have hypoglycemia. My fasting blood sugar was 60, and by the time they took my five-hour test it was down to 35. My doctor says that's quite low."

Her companion listened quietly to her story, then said, "The trouble with my doctor is that he doesn't worry enough about me. I've been nervous for years. He has never taken a blood sugar test. He just says, 'It's your nerves,' and lets it go at that. Next time I see him I'm going to ask about my blood sugar. If he laughs it off, I'll go to your doctor instead."

Pill Poppers

I call it pill popping when people take medicines as nonchalantly as they swallow candy. There's a tendency to make one's own distinctions between what are "strong" medicines and what are "harmless" ones. For example, consider this patient's complaint about her husband's penchant for taking pills.

"My husband worries me. Every day he takes aspirin by the handful (at least a dozen aspirin a day). He has headaches. The doctor has found no reason except tension. Once he told him to take an aspirin or two for relief. Now, as I said, he takes too many.

"He says, 'What's the commotion? I get headaches, and aspirin helps them. It's a harmless medicine. What's wrong in taking a dozen aspirin? They give me relief. That's all I care about.'

"I'm really concerned about him because I've heard that even harmless medicines sometimes can be dangerous. Is it true that aspirin can cause bleeding from the stomach? I'm afraid that someday he will have a hemorrhage."

I said, "It's true that your husband is a pill popper. In his case, apparently harmless aspirin is the staff he leans on. Other people may pop tranquilizers or sedatives or sleeping pills or iron tablets or vitamins. All apparently harmless, but all potentially dangerous if taken in doses that are too large and for overly long periods of time.

"It is true that aspirin is one of the wonder drugs. It brings relief to millions. Between twenty and thirty tons are consumed daily in the United States for various aches and pains. But too few people realize that aspirin sometimes can cause bleeding from the stomach or intestines, and that it may be bad for ulcer patients and for those who suffer from asthma and other allergic conditions.

"Mind you, I'm not trying to downgrade aspirin, which I consider one of our most useful drugs. I'm just warning your husband and others that pill popping may be dangerous even when apparently harmless drugs are swallowed."

A week later her husband, a tense, self-sufficient individual, came to the office. He said, "What's this I hear about the dangers of aspirin? My wife's been on me to come and hear what you told her."

I repeated the story, examined him, and found sufficient reason in his history to suggest that he take a glucose tolerance test. It was unquestionably low. After being on a diet practically free from sweets, his headaches gradually diminished and disappeared. End of a pill popper.

Food Misconceptions

Undoubtedly, a common cause of headaches is diets that are far from normal. A headache often disappears quickly when a little food overcomes a hungry period. For years you have heard, "Have a headache? Perhaps you're hungry.

Better take some food." We know, unscientifically, that the system needs something to get rid of the headache, but we are completely unaware that the culprit may be hypoglycemia.

However, food and headaches are often horses in tandem that pull in opposite directions. Too many people eat in a way that brings daily insult to the blood sugar content, and the consequences they suffer are headaches and any of the scores of other complaints I have already mentioned.

"Frankly, I'm confused! About diets that is! One weight reduction diet calls for two eggs every morning, cheeses, and other high protein foods. Another diet says that if you start each meal with grapefruit or grapefruit juice it tends to eat up the fat, and you can eat as much food as you want. The grapefruit is supposed to be a catalyst. And another diet is so skimpy that you wonder how you can get through the day on it.

"I could go on mentioning the various diets I have received from friends who say, 'This is the Mayo Clinic diet,' or, 'This is a very special diet I got from a friend.'

"In trying several of these diets I was afraid that eating too many eggs would produce high cholesterol, that eating too many tomatoes or taking too much tomato juice would cause acidity, and that too much grapefruit also would cause a breaking out and itchiness. And the starvation diets gave me terrific headaches and made me terribly nervous.

"What I'm concerned about is this: I'm only in my early thirties and would like to be around a little longer—without these headaches. What foods does one require each day for good health? If we omit bread, is this bad? If we refrain from eggs, are we depriving ourselves of necessary protein? I'm driving my husband crazy. I wish that once and for all someone would come out with the facts of daily requirements needed for good health. I feel that many adults, as well as children, are so food conscious that they are probably suffering from malnutrition because of constant dieting. What is your theory?"

I told her not to take it too personally when I said that she was too food conscious and that she was a ripe condidate for the ever-increasing army of food faddists who are afraid to eat this and too scared to eat that.

"When you come right down to it," I said, "eating a healthful diet should really be a natural and easy part of decision making in your life. For example, what's more natural than to drink when you are thirsty and eat when you are hungry? The fact is that most of us eat what is good for us; otherwise, we wouldn't survive. But some people, including you, get on these diet kicks, which throw the wrench into their eating machinery."

People are too gullible about food requirements. Fads and ads contribute to the confusion. I believe that the quickest way to become confused about what and what not to eat is to open an ear to what friends say, to what faddists say, to what advertisements say. If you do, you will believe that molasses and yogurt will guarantee a ripe old age, that mixing ice cream and seafood at the same meal is poisonous, that fish is really brain food. (One of the stupidest men I know eats fish seven days a week.)

I told this patient that she needed only a well-rounded and satisfactory diet—suitable portions of proteins, fats, carbohydrates, minerals, and vitamins in her daily intake of edibles. "From now on," I said, "take your diet formulas from one source—me. That will save you from faddists, advertisements, and well-meaning friends. Besides, since you've been starving yourself lately let's be sure that your headaches are not due to hypoglycemia."

She refused to undergo the blood sugar tolerance test because "I have an ungodly fear of needles." Nevertheless, the therapeutic test indicated that she was a likely member of the low blood sugar group. Within one week after she began a sensible diet and frequent snacks, she said, "A curtain has lifted. I haven't had a headache since the first day I cut down on sweets and began to eat sensibly."

Headache in Children

Many parents find it hard to believe that the headaches their young children suffer are real and not excuses for misdemeanors. Many a youngster suffers headaches in solitude. He is completely misunderstood. Not only does he have the headache to contend with but he also has a parent who is punitive—one who spanks him and thinks of him as a neurotic.

"What can a mother do with a five-year-old boy who becomes obstreperous and complains of headaches? I've tried everything from being nice to giving him a good spanking. Otherwise, he seems healthy. He has had his tonsils out and his sinuses appear to be normal. I think I must have a young neurotic on my hands."

I said, "I can't even guess what's wrong, but I can imagine your frustration. And your child's. Therefore, the first suggestion I have to make is that you discontinue the spankings. If you have ever had a bad headache yourself, I doubt that you would welcome that kind of therapy.

"I will try a guess or two, though. Have you ever considered the possibility that your child is allergic or possibly suffers from low blood sugar? I believe that these problems are commonly overlooked as causes of headaches in youngsters as well as in adults."

I recall one "obstreperous" little boy who became a sweet, easily manageable child after the discovery that he was allergic to tomatoes. No more tomatoes, no more headaches and irritability.

Then there was the little girl who became depressed and wouldn't go out to play because "I've got a headache, mother." She, too, was considered a budding neurotic until her doctor deleted chocolate from her diet. He also found that her allergy was complicated by an abnormally low blood sugar. Proper treatment transformed her from a "neurotic" to a normal little girl.

Headaches, nervousness, and depression can come on within hours after the offending food is consumed, and these symptoms may last a day or longer. Common offenders in the diet are corn, tomatoes, citrus fruits, chocolate, eggs, wheat, milk, fish, nuts. Sometimes vitamins or other medications will set off headaches like a time bomb.

The point I want to stress is that if foods are not found to be the triggering element then it is wise not to overlook an abnormally low blood sugar. Better take the youngster to your pediatrician and possibly to an allergist. Remember that most children with headaches are not neurotics; something real probably is "bugging" them. A parent's job, and responsibility, is to be patient rather than mistrusting with a child.

Advice from Headache Specialists

In *Headaches*, Noah D. Fabricant, M.D., of Chicago, wrote:

Hypoglycemia causes headaches in some people. Hypoglycemic headaches characteristically occur before meals, after exercise, during a period of starvation, and as the result of an overdose of insulin taken for diabetes. . . .In general, hypoglycemia is characterized by extreme hunger. Happily, the treatment for this condition is easy to carry out; headaches are relieved by food in the form of frequent, small feedings.

In his introduction to *Help for Your Headache* by Edward Edelson, Seymour Diamond, M.D., co-director of the Headache Clinic, Mt. Sinai Hospital and Medical Center in New York, writes, "The detective ability of a Sherlock Holmes may be necessary in some instances to find the key to the headache problem." These words underline what I have said a number of times.

Later in the book Edelson shows the relationship between headache and hypoglycemia.

> In most normal people, hypoglycemia will occur only when something prevents an adequate intake of food. That "something" could be a skipped meal or two. Or it could be brought on by one of the crash diets that weight-conscious Americans are apt to try in an effort to take off a few pounds quickly. . . . Hypoglycemia produces weakness and trembling, with a dull headache that seems to suffuse the entire head, and a quite natural feeling of hunger. Eating usually eliminates the headaches and the other symptoms. *If a good meal doesn't work, then it's time for a visit to the doctor to see whether hyperinsulinism—overproduction of insulin—is to blame.* [Italics mine.]

Finding the Causes

The qualities of a Sherlock Holmes are indeed necessary to successfully investigate and overcome chronic headache, because headache is only a symptom, not a disease. There's trouble somewhere. How and where to find it? Think of all the possibilities that must be considered and then perhaps discarded before the real reason is discovered.

Are the headaches due to tension, the most common cause of headaches? I call it the Big T. Whether you are an executive in a large corporation or a manager of a small shop or office, your body and mind may suffer the effects of tension and fatigue in the form of headaches and other serious complications. You may have family problems that you have been unwilling to reveal because you are ashamed. The true source of tension headache may be a wife, a husband, children, boss, co-workers—anyone with whom you have frequent contact.

Will an eyeglass fitting or treatment of an ear condition solve the problem? Is the headache a vascular type of the migraine variety? Is it due to muscle contraction at the back of the neck? (Then simple massage often is effective.) Are the sinuses, teeth, or nose at fault? Is it a cluster (histamine) headache? Is it due to hypertension or heart disease, arthritis in the cervical spine, infection, allergy, or actual trouble in the brain? Is it a consequence of infectious disease elsewhere in the body—influenza, for example?

I mention this long list of etiological factors in headaches so that you will not believe that a high protein, low carbohydrate diet is the sure antidote for your own headache. The true cause must be found, and your doctor must know *all* the facts in order to find it.

But I repeat: if both you and your doctor have been frustrated in your search, if relief has not been found, neither you nor he should overlook the possibility that hypoglycemia may be a factor. Even if it is only a marginal contributor to your discomforts, proper treatment of low blood sugar will help in the management of headache.

There is no substitute for complete knowledge. And no investigation is complete if it overlooks the possibility that hypoglycemia may be the prime reason for headache.

8

Irregularities in Normal Hearts

MORE people suffer from imaginary heart trouble than from actual heart disease. (Note the distinction between trouble and actual disease.) Only those who believe that this symptom or that presages an early demise know what it is to fear that every day may be the last.

Skips and Palpitations

"By present-day standards, I am still young—only thirty-four. I have four children, a fine husband, and a lovely home. But all this adds up to nothing, a big zero, when you're afraid you'll leave this earthly heaven any day because you're sure you have a weak heart.

"My trouble is palpitation and skips. A half-dozen fine cardiologists have examined me carefully, and all have come up with a diagnosis of nervous heart! They could find nothing wrong. Yet I still keep getting the skips. Whenever I do, I feel the end is near. My heart seems to turn over in my throat. When I lie in bed at night, I have all I can do not to wake my husband and tell him to call the doctor. In between skips (sometimes for days or even weeks) I'm still scared. I'm afraid that they'll return. And they do. Is there any hope for me?"

I went carefully into her history. She admitted that she was a two-pack-a-day smoker, liked two or three highballs before dinner, and was a skimpy eater. When the skips came on, she felt jittery and trembly "way down deep inside," which made her feel that she was going to pass out.

My examination, like those of the six cardiologists she had consulted, was negative, although there was an occasional premature contraction (skipped heart beat). X rays, electrocardiograms, and physical examination revealed no evidence of cardiac disease.

I said, "Look. You are one of at least 15 million Americans who are anxious about their normal hearts. They also live in an anxiety state, fearful that the end is near. Like you, many do not believe their doctors when they are told that they do not have real heart disease. They may, like you, have skips and palpitations. Or they may complain of shortness of breath, occasional swollen ankles, or fleeting pains in the left chest. Yet doctors must make the diagnosis of cardiac neurosis rather than of actual disease.

"I have found that after many months or years people who suffer from imaginary heart trouble at last learn to believe their doctors are right. Simply being alive begins to make an impression on them. They realize that if they were as bad as they thought, they would have been dead long ago.

"You'll have to learn to believe your doctors. These days they do not hesitate to tell you if you have actual heart disease. Be thankful that you have been given a not-guilty verdict by six cardiologists.

"But see here. You've admitted that the other doctors also suggested that you stop smoking—and you haven't. If you expect to improve, you'll have to make a contribution to your own improvement. Quit! And there's something else. I'm making an appointment for you to have a six-hour glucose tolerance test. A single fasting blood sugar doesn't tell us everything we want to know."

She agreed, threw her pack of cigarettes in my waste-basket, and never smoked again. Her blood sugar tolerance test showed definite evidence that she had hypoglycemia. Within a few weeks after she began a high protein, low carbohydrate diet, and also cut down on alcohol and eliminated coffee, she had lost most of her anxiety. Although her heart skips continued for a few months longer, she did not complain that she was in danger of dying.

"Somehow," she said, "I feel more courageous, less jittery, and stronger—at home and when I'm out socially. Do you suppose it could all be due to my new diet? Is that the possible answer?"

"Probable, not possible," I said.

Rapid Beat

"My heart often runs away with itself. It feels like horses' hooves pounding on a racetrack. I'll be sitting quietly and boom! It's off, racing away anywhere from one to five minutes. It's a horrible, scary feeling. Then it stops—I mean beats more slowly—as if nothing had happened. I've been too scared to come and find out why."

For no apparent reason (although it often occurs in anxious persons), the heart races like mad and then suddenly reverts to normal. Some people have daily attacks, others only every few weeks or months. Some attacks last longer than five minutes—for days, even weeks.

Pressing hard on the carotid nerve in the neck often will shorten the attack, as will some medicines. What's important is learning the true diagnosis. Sometimes a fast, irregular heartbeat develops when a thyroid gland is overactive. Such auricular fibrillation is also sometimes a complication of a rheumatic, arteriosclerotic, or hypertensive heart. Coronary artery disease may weaken a heart muscle and cause it to be irritable.

But the important thing to remember is that there are all kinds of runaway hearts. Sometimes they are healthy hearts. Cutting out tobacco, liquor, and caffeine and taking tranquilizers will help. Even when the heart is diseased, medications are available to rein it in so that it won't beat so fast.

After reassurance, this patient seemed to feel better about her heart. Nevertheless, I prescribed tranquilizers, made an appointment for her to have blood sugar studies made, and saw her again in about two weeks. She had a flat curve; yet minor modification in her carbohydrate intake had lessened her anxiety.

I followed her progress for at least five years. During that time she had only two minor incidents in which her horse "pounded down the track." As she said, "I rarely go to the races any more."

Chest Pains

One woman, evidently nervous and worried about her husband, asked me if there was any need to be concerned that his left chest pains might be due to heart disease. He officiated during the football and basketball seasons and was a full-time government worker as well. The pains in his chest seemed to come on when work pressured him or when he was tired. During his examination, the family doctor said the electrocardiograms were all right; the pain was due to muscle spasm and to the food the man ate, such as pizza. He took digitalis pills when the pain got bad.

I told her that making a diagnosis is like solving a mystery. When symptoms (clues) don't seem to fit into the puzzle, the medical detective begins to wonder whether or not he is on the right track.

"For example," I said, "in your husband's case the pieces don't appear to fit. If, as your doctor says, your husband's heart is normal, why is he taking digitalis? Either it is or it isn't heart disease. If it isn't, most doctors do not prescribe a heart medicine for a patient with a normal heart. If it is, then either the doctor or your husband is withholding the true condition. I believe that when heart disease or any other ailment is present the patient and his family should know the truth. Otherwise, it is impossible to have the patient's full cooperation."

I told her that angina pectoris can be present though the electrocardiograms are normal. Another clue didn't fit into the puzzle. In my experience, most left-sided chest pains are not caused by heart disease.

Subsequent examination confirmed my suspicion. His heart was all right; but his diet was for the birds. A sensible diet neutralized his anxiety and reduced his chest pains. Low blood sugar combined with strenuous work had given him undue anxiety about his heart. He had a flat sugar curve.

Often patients who suffer from imaginary heart trouble become completely frustrated. They do not know where to turn next. They have become dizzy from traveling on the medical merry-go-around.

"I am in desperate need of some medical advice. I hope that you will find time to give it to me. My problem is that for approximately four months I have been having periodic pains and tightness in my chest. The pains seem to be of a fleeting nature in different areas. However, once in a while they hang on for longer periods. They are just as likely to come on at night as during the day.

"I am thirty-eight years old, six feet tall, and a thin 145 pounds. I have been physically active all my life, but now I hesitate to take part in sports like tennis and golf.

"I first saw a doctor about these pains four months ago, after I was kept awake most of one night with a constant pain directly under my breastbone. ECGs showed that my heart was all right. An upper GI series was also negative.

"I've gone to three doctors, and none have been able to convince me that I am not sick. I've only been accused of worrying too much about myself. They look at me as if I were a moron simply because I ask questions about myself. Believe me, the only thing I worry about is not knowing what's wrong with me! I feel that I am entitled to know everything there is to know about myself. But they don't give me more than a few minutes, and even then they don't seem to listen. Will you give me the time to tell what's bothering me?"

I set aside an hour for just that—listening. What I learned was why he was so thin and so worried. His eating habits were atrocious. He had suddenly decided to become a vegetarian, without even learning its principles. He was protein-starved. His blood sugar curve was flat. He was suffering from hypoglycemia.

Like the others whose case histories I have described, his "heart symptons" practically disappeared after he began to eat sensibly. It was as easy as all that. I do not recall having a more thankful patient. And think of it. All I had used in treatment was a mixture of big ears (mine) and a sensible diet (his).

Am I too diet oriented? Do I believe that diet, like magic,

is the cure for all aches and pains and worries? Of course not. But I'd rather accept such an accusation than be guilty of overlooking deficient or lopsided diets as the possible cause of much unnecessary suffering.

9

Hypoglycemia's Relationship to Other Diseases

Ulcer

Ulcer often is found in the most unsuspected patients. This unhappy patient came for treatment for what she considered to be an uncomplicated obesity problem.

"I'm having marital problems because of my excessive weight. I tip the scales at about 250 pounds, as you will see. My husband says that if I could weigh about 130, my weight before marriage, everything would be OK. He says I'm not the same girl he married, and I admit I'm not.

"I've been on diets of my own, but I've failed to lose. My husband says, 'Why do you eat so much?' When I tell him I eat when I get angry or upset or tense, he says, 'You must be mad an awful lot.'

"This didn't help. Funny, yes, but no answer for me. In addition to being fat, I'm tired all the time. I also have been

79

having pains in my stomach when it's empty. I mean in midmorning and midafternoon, and sometimes they wake me around 2 A.M.

"I can't seem to stay on a diet. It's no joke. You know, you can be an alcoholic and people still love you. You can be a drug user and people will sympathize and understand. But if you're fat, it's all your fault! Everyone laughs. Nobody, especially your own husband, understands what you're going through. Nobody seems to love someone who is fat. It isn't true that everyone loves the fat one.

"I hope you can save my marriage. I've thought of leaving home, kids, and husband, but I know that isn't the solution."

For years, she had been using a "do-it-yourself kit" in trying to solve her problem. Some people are successful in treating obesity without the help of a doctor; in fact, most are. But in her case, it was important that she consult a medical man, because studies showed that obesity was not her only problem.

X rays revealed a large duodenal ulcer, and blood sugar curves indicated that her constant desire for sweets was due to hypoglycemia. The more she ate, the more her ulcer was upset, and the fatter she became. Ulcer and hypoglycemia are often associated. Both often cause similar symptoms. For example, her early morning pains might well have been due to a very low blood sugar, which often occurs at that time.

Under careful guidance and sympathetic management (to make up for all the months of frustration and misunderstanding), her weight came down to 160, and her ulcer came under control. So did her husband.

Allergy

One estimate is that at least twenty million Americans suffer from some type of allergy. It may occur at any age. A baby in its crib may have a skin eruption because of a milk sensitivity; a teenager may have a penicillin reaction; a middle-aged businessman may get stomach upsets from eating chocolate; an elderly woman may wheeze because of asthma.

An allergy is simply a sensitivity to ordinarily harmless substances. These substances are called allergens. They can be swallowed or inhaled, or they can cause irritation by actual contact or by injection.

Here are some common sources of allergic disease:

Inhalants-pollens from weeds, trees, grasses, and plants, dust, mold spores, animal danders, hair lotion, feathers, cosmetics, insecticide sprays, chemicals, and tobacco.

Food-fruits, nuts, fish, eggs, milk, wheat, beans, and others.

Contactants-insecticides, drugs, resins, cosmetics, dyes, rubber, fabrics, metals, plastics, foliage.

Drugs by injection or by mouth-serums, antibiotics, insulin, liver extract, hormones.

Bacteria-germs in nose, throat, tonsils, bronchial tubes, ears, sinuses, and other areas of the body.

Thousands of persons suffer needlessly from allergy because they never think of that possibility. "It's only a cold." "It's indigestion." "It's bronchitis." Whenever you are plagued by symptoms that are mysterious and do not fit into any proper diagnostic niche, you and your doctor should consider the possibility of allergy. Why suffer from itch, cough, headaches, indigestion—or worse—when there may be a cure for the asking?

Treatment of allergy is either *active* or *passive*. Active treatment builds up the body's resistance to allergens by means of steadily increasing desensitization doses by injection to control reactions to ragweed, dust, molds, and other irritants.

Passive treatment is like coming out of the rain. The patient tries to get away from the sensitizing agents by giving up certain elements in the diet, moving elsewhere (which invariably doesn't help), or living in a house that is as dust free as possible.

"I have an allergic boy. He was constantly hungry. But I mean ravenous! At times he couldn't wait to get at food because of actual hunger pains. He was sensitive to ragweed, and the doctor was trying to desensitize him, but it didn't work out well. All measures failed.

"The allergist said there was danger that Freddie might go into asthma attacks. I'd heard somewhere that a low blood sugar may sometimes cause these hungry feelings, so the doctor was willing to send him to a laboratory for a blood sugar test. The curve was low. They said it was hypoglycemia. He was put on a strict diet, and within a few months he was better, even though it was still the height of the hay fever season. The near-asthma attacks disappeared. So did his hunger pains."

Experiments have shown that allergic reactions may be made worse by low blood sugar. In one study, about 25 percent of asthmatic patients were hypoglycemic. When the low blood sugar was treated, the asthma improved. (In fact, some asthmatics improve when they develop diabetes.) There is something about a higher blood sugar that seems to protect against allergy. For example, it is well known that diabetics are not so likely to get allergic involvements as are those with normal blood sugar.

Rheumatic Heart Disease

In the 1940's, while making rounds on my medical service at McCook Memorial Hospital in Hartford, Connecticut, I examined quite a few youngsters who were being treated for rheumatic heart disease. At the time I postulated: If it's true that the high blood sugar of diabetic patients seems to protect them from such diseases as rheumatic fever and the complication of heart disease, is it possible that the blood sugar levels in these children are low?

I ordered glucose tolerance curves, and in the first ten or eleven patients, as I recall, I discovered that the blood sugar curves were low. (I reported this study in *The Journal of the American Medical Association.*) At the time, I was not aware that the proper treatment of these patients was a low carbohydrate, high protein diet. Like most doctors then, I believed that the best way to bring up the blood sugar was to prescribe sweets.

Now, we recognize the fallacy of such management. We know that the more sugar the patient takes, the more insulin he secretes, and the lower the blood sugar falls. More recent reports have indicated that children with a history of rheumatic fever were spared future attacks and heart complications because they had been on high protein, low carbohydrate diets—especially when blood sugar studies had indicated the presence of hypoglycemia.

Thyroid Disease

Diagnosis is relatively easy in an out-and-out attack of gallstone colic, in typical acute appendicitis, or in a full-blown pneumonia. In scores of other conditions, typical symptoms and signs point their accusing fingers at the suspect.

But some cases of gallbladder disease, appendicitis, or pneumonia are overlooked because they are atypical. One condition often unsuspected is an underfunctioning thyroid gland, or *hypothyroidism*.

She was a sixty-two-year-old housewife—overweight, skin dry, hair thinning and falling out, always tired and sleepy, always chilly, no ambition. "I let my house and husband go. Just sat around trying to regain my energy. Took all kinds of vitamins and iron tablets, but there was no improvement. I was tired, dejected, and nervous. People called me a dull companion, and I realized I was."

Blood tests showed that her trouble was in the thyroid gland. A daily dosage of thyroid extract tablets was prescribed, but in spite of her cooperation she had not improved after three months of medication. She was still nervous and tense, and her husband labeled her "nothing more than a psychoneurotic."

After more months of thyroid medication, repeated blood tests for thyroid activity showed that it had come back to normal. Where else to look?

The trouble was hypoglycemia. She continued to take thyroid extract, but she also rearranged her diet to include the proper amounts of proteins and vitamins—and gave up her excessive coffee drinking and high carbohydrate consumption. Improvement followed almost within days, and her husband has willingly removed the tag "psychoneurotic."

Alcoholism

I try to feel charitable toward people who continue to judge others who are at the mercy of alcohol as if they were immoral rather than just plain sick. No matter how often experts appear on radio or television, or write about chronic alcoholism in magazines, books, and newspaper articles, there are bound to be those who still look down their noses at chronic alcoholics. A favorite expression is "He's nothing but an old sot." Not only do they disparage the moral values of the person caught in the tentacles of alcoholism, but they also refuse to believe (or remember) that this affliction is really a disease.

You might expect such an obtuse observation from one

who is a teetotaler, but it doesn't benefit the person who is proud of being able to "take a few" without letting alcohol interfere with social or business obligations. Yet many such individuals do not realize that they themselves walk the tightrope between social drinking and alcoholism. Many of the millions of so-called social drinkers are closer to the edge than they realize.

These people wake up in the morning to a glass of the stuff they had the night before. They take a midmorning drink. They imbibe a few martinis or a couple of beers at lunch. Midafternoon is the time for refueling. And at night they take three to four fingers of scotch or bourbon. True, they haven't yet earned the label "old sot," but they may be closer than they think. Social drinkers should beware; they should take inventory.

"What is being done about alcoholism? We hear of drives for the management of epilepsy, heart disease, tuberculosis, and all the others. What about alcoholism?

"I'm the wife of a chronic alcoholic. Can you imagine how it feels to be forgotten? Why doesn't the government do something to help? Haven't people yet gotten around to realizing that the chronic alcoholic is sick and not a criminal?"

There is good reason for this woman's note of despair. The wheels grind slowly. However, the government finally is taking a hand. At last we are facing alcoholism as a problem that requires solution. It's about time when we consider that five to six million Americans are alcoholics. If you drink, the chances are one in fifteen that you, too, are an alcoholic. Even if you are a teetotaler, the chances are one in five that you have a close relative who is an alcoholic.

According to the U.S. Department of Health, Education, and Welfare, alcoholism today ranks as the nation's fourth largest health hazard behind heart disease, mental illness, and cancer. Alcoholics have a death rate 2.5 times higher than the national average. Records of public (nonfederal) mental hospitals indicate that in the early 1960's 15 percent of total admissions were alcoholics. Half of all annual non-traffic arrests in the United States are for drunkenness. These 2 million arrests (in 1965) not only burden law enforcement officials but also crowd the courts, jails, and workhouses. Most of these arrests for intoxication are repeaters and hardcore alcoholics. National Safety Council studies estimate that drinking is a factor in about 50 percent of the nation's fatal traffic accidents and in from 13 to 15 percent of nonfatal accidents.

No investigator yet has discovered the actual cause or specific cure for alcoholism. However, I offer the suggestion that many alcoholics might be benefited if some active measures were taken to try to rearrange their daily diets. The main complaint of onlookers (family and friends) is that "he's starving himself; he hardly eats, just drinks."

In depriving themselves of proper nutrition, alcoholics invite actual brain and liver damage that in many instances may have been prevented. It is not surprising that when blood sugar readings were taken in alcoholics a flat or abnormally low sugar tolerance was discovered.

Which came first, the chicken or the egg? Did hypoglycemia induce drinking? Or did alcoholism produce the low blood sugar? Whichever the association, undoubtedly the treatment of hypoglycemia by means of a high protein diet and sufficient vitamins in many instances has given the patient the strength to undergo treatment for alcoholism.

However, the treatment of hypoglycemia should not be considered a cure but a reinforcement. The truly hypoglycemic alcoholic is not physically strong enough either to recognize the disease or to "take the cure."

10

Doctor-Patient Relations

Being healthy is a natural state; hence many of the complex and wondrous accomplishments of the body are taken for granted. For example, the stomach is ready to digest anything and everything you plop into it; the heart beats every waking and sleeping moment of your entire lifetime; the brain gives you the sense for accomplishment, enjoyment, and self-preservation; the legs carry you; the arms hold; the kidneys excrete poisonous material and waste; the liver manufactures and stores many life-giving substances; the glands give you zest and purpose; your reproductive organs help to create new life.

But one day something happens. The finely tuned organism called the body goes out of whack. Something falters somewhere. When that something is blood sugar metabolism, the patient soon knows that something is wrong. Many un-

happy innocents crawl rather than skip through life because low blood sugar is overlooked. They are shut off
from normal intercourse with their fellows, like people cast
off after shipwreck and bypassed daily by those who might
rescue them.

The Need for Physical Checkups

Everyone has had a horrible nightmare at some time in
life. Will you ever forget the sense of relief when you woke
up? Imagination turns into reality, and things aren't possibly
so bad as they were only a few moments ago. For many
anxious and nervous people, a medical checkup with a verdict of not-guilty acts the same way.

I have examined thousands of scared people. Their sta-
tions in life did not matter. They ranged from office boys
to presidents of corporations. Each had a secret fear that
even their best friends, and perhaps their own families, didn't
suspect.

I recall one man who was so nervous that he limped
through life for years before gathering the courage to have
a complete physical. He had complained of frequent heart
palpitations and was certain that his end was near. When
he learned that his nervousness and palpitations were due to
hypoglycemia, he actually did a hop, skip, and jump in the
office.

"What a fool I've been," he said. "The fear of having a bad
heart has colored every waking moment of my existence
for the past few years."

One woman was certain that she would someday be a
mental case. A long talk after a complete physical examination convinced her that there was no relationship between
her future mental health and the fact that her father (over
seventy-five) was in an institution because of some brain

trouble. Two weeks later, after beginning a high protein diet for her recently discovered hypoglycemia, she said, "I feel so much better. What a fool I've been to suffer so long without reason. For years, I've been afraid to come in for a checkup because I was sure you would find some evidence of weakness in my nervous system."

If you have any doubts whatever about your health, don't live in unnecessary anxiety. See your doctor. You'll get a great lift from a physical checkup.

One patient told me, "When I'm on my way to your office, I resolve that I'm going to tell you everything that's on my mind. But when I get here, I'm transformed into an entirely different person. I clam up. I have trouble telling you the complete truth about myself. I realize that keeping my problems to myself will never do me any good. I say to myself, 'Get rid of your repressions. Tell everything that's on your mind.' But most of the time I leave feeling that my visit hasn't been entirely well spent. I know it isn't your fault; it's mine."

Consider another patient who said, "I admit I'm a peculiar sort of patient. I never felt entirely satisfied after an office visit. I know the reason. I forced you to play guessing games with me. I was like the patient in the joke who went to his dentist with a toothache. The dentist asked him, 'Which tooth hurts?' and the patient answered, 'You tell me! You're the dentist!'

"I was the same way with you. I came to your office, paid your nurse after taking your valuable time away from other sick patients, but I never really told you what bothered me. Not until later.   .

"Do you remember the day when you asked me how I sleep? I said fine! The truth was that I hadn't slept more than four full hours a night for months. That was reason enough for my tiredness. You, poor man, kept looking for clues. Then you asked me if I ever felt nervous and trembly in midafternoon. I said yes. And you said, 'I'm sending you to the laboratory next week for a sugar tolerance test.' And that was it. Since then, I've felt fine. That's why I have the courage now to confess about what a bad patient I've been."

It bears repetition; when you go to your doctor come clean. No matter what your complaints, whatever your fears, divulge them. Come out in the open. He won't laugh at you or ridicule you. If you can possibly take him into your confidence, do so. He won't judge you on a moral basis; you have nothing to be ashamed of. The surest hope for well-being is to state your fears out loud and not keep them to yourself.

The Importance of Early Diagnosis

"Whenever I feel sick," the patient said, "even though I get very uncomfortable, I hesitate to bother you. I figure that with so many really sick people who need attention it isn't fair to you and to them to take up precious time. Besides, I don't want the label 'hypochondriac' pinned on me. Don't you think I deserve some kind of medal instead?"

I told her that I both agreed and disagreed. People shouldn't go running to their doctors for every little ache and pain. But the trouble comes in taking on yourself the responsibility of deciding what is little and what is big. At times, even serious illness masquerades as something trifling and not a threat to health and life.

If you put off a visit simply because you feel silly and are afraid of the hypochondriac tag, then you may actually be endangering your life.

It's better to chance being called a hypochondriac, see your doctor a few extra times during the year, and be safe rather than take it on yourself to distinguish between unimportant symptoms and serious disease. Doctors do appreciate patients who come early enough so that disease can be cured. We hate to say, "If you had only come in to see me a few months earlier." Do not feel that you are bothering your doctor in trying to establish the presence or absence of serious illness.

The term hypochondriac should not be used loosely. Most people are normally apprehensive, not hypochondriacal. Both doctor and patient have a mutual responsibility not to resort to this classification. Sick people want to get well; so it is natural for some to exaggerate their symptoms.

A doctor's relationship with his patient often hangs by a slender cord. A doctor who uses a descriptive phrase such as "It's only your nerves" often snaps the confidence that has been built up over the years. I do not believe that it should be used to describe the reason for any person's suffering. Nor do I believe that a really tactful physician would use the word hypochondriac as a descriptive tag.

Of course, it is true that many people make unnecessary visits to the doctor. They admit that the only reason they go is to have the doctor tell them what they already know. One says, "I know I'm fat and need to lose weight. And I know how to do it. But it makes me feel better to have the doctor tell me. It gives me a shove into doing what I should."

Another says, "I'll bet you ten to one that he'll tell me I'm smoking too much for my own good. I know it without going to the doctor. But when I hear it from the horse's (pardon me) mouth, perhaps I'll really do something about quitting."

Human nature doesn't change. I have been reading what Michel de Montaigne said in his autobiography about his relationship with doctors. "When I am sick, I send for them if they are near at hand, merely to have their company; and I pay them as others do. I give them leave to order me to keep myself warm, for I like to do it anyway. I let them recommend leeks or lettuce for my soup, put me on white wine or claret, or anything else that is indifferent to my taste and habits."

"I am a forty-five-year-old housewife, and my chief complaint is headache. I've gone to my doctor, and without any kind of examination he has labeled my trouble tension headache. What I can't understand is how a doctor can make that diagnosis without at least giving you an examination. I'm not any better. What shall I do?"

Ask for consultation. If refused, you have the right to change doctors. This abrupt and unequivocal reply is my reaction whenever any diagnosis whatever is made without talking to a patient, listening, or laying a diagnostic hand on him. Doctors are not little gods who can look at you and tell you what's wrong just like that.

11

Diets for Hypoglycemics

ONCE your doctor has made the diagnosis of functional hypoglycemia, practically the entire responsibility for your well-being depends on you. The methodology is easy to explain but often difficult to follow. As normal human beings, it is difficult for us to change our diet patterns. Sweets are a universal temptation.

If your blood sugar is chronically low, there are foods you must avoid like the plague. I'll list these first so that you are fully warned. (As you have learned, your purpose will be to protect the islets of Langerhans in your pancreas from oversecreting insulin and causing the abrupt fall in blood sugar.)

Reject:

Beer, cordials, cocktails, wines.

Caffeine-in ordinary coffee, strong tea, and cold beverages.

Sugar, honey, candies, cakes, pies, puddings, and custards, ice cream, pastries.

Macaroni, spaghetti, potatoes, noodles, large portions of bread.

Raisins, grapes, plums, bananas, dates, figs.

Soft drinks, colas, and any other drinks sweetened with sugar, chocolate, cocoa, canned fruits in syrup, prune juice, grape juice.

Pizza, crackers, rice, doughnuts.

Accept:

Vegetables-asparagus, broccoli, avocado, cabbage, brussels sprouts, celery, carrots, cucumbers, corn, cauliflower, tomatoes, eggplant, squash, turnips, string beans, peas, onions, radishes.

Fruits-grapefruit, oranges, tangerines, lemons, peaches, apples, pears, berries.

Drinks-decaffeinated coffee, weak tea, coffee substitutes sweetened with saccharin, club soda, distilled liquors.

Proteins-meats, fish, poultry, cheese, eggs, milk.

Such is the spare outline, the ribs, the steel superstructure of the hypoglycemic diet. Each individual will require personal counseling by his doctor; the variety and amount of foods will be dependent on the patient's weight and general health. Vitamin B complex and other vitamins and medications will be added as required.

If you are hypoglycemic you must learn to eat by the clock. Time must not go by unheeded. If you are forgetful, wear a miniature alarm to warn you that it's time for a snack or a meal. "Three squares" are no longer for you.

Six to eight small meals are preferable. Large meals make too insistent demands on the insulin-producing pancreas, thereby causing wide swings in blood sugar. Several small meals call for less sudden insulin production and more uneventful carbohydrate metabolism.

Meal regulation calls for a change in habit pattern. Everyone knows that bad habits, like a reluctant dragon, can be overcome only with determination. Patients say, "I forget to eat often."

Especially is this true for the one accustomed to no breakfast at all or only black coffee and cake, no lunch or another coffee and sweet roll, and a heavy dinner early in the evening. (I call this the dog diet, a once-a-day gulping of food and drink.) "I can't face food in the morning" will have to be replaced by "I've learned to enjoy a good breakfast of fruit juice, cereal, bacon and eggs, a slice of toast, and weak tea."

Here is a working schedule that can be the basis for your change in diet habits so that your blood sugar will not plummet and rise like an elevator gone crazy, thereby giving you all the hypoglycemic symptoms as it suddenly falls below normal.

When you arise: 4 ounces of fruit juice or half a grapefruit.

Breakfast (Breaking an approximately ten-hour fast): grapefruit or juice, bacon (or ham) and egg(s), one slice of bread, butter, beverage.

Midmorning: 4 ounces of juice.

Lunch: fish, meat, or fowl; large servings of salad with mayonnaise or French dressing; one slice of bread; fruit for dessert; beverage.

Midafternoon: 8 ounces of milk, cheese snacks, or nuts.

Dinner: soup, meat (fish or poultry) vegetables, one slice of bread, beverage, dessert.

Every two hours until bedtime: milk or snacks.

12

Diets for Nonhypoglycemics

Patients with confessed bad diet habits often ask, "Suppose tests show that I don't have low blood sugar? I realize I haven't been eating right. Will you give me some food fundamentals so I can understand how to go about changing my eating habits?"

I have had many sources to choose from, but none, I think, offers simpler and more suitable information than the U.S. Department of Agriculture in its leaflet No. 424, *Food for Fitness (A Daily Food Guide.)*

Each day food should supply you with many different nutrients: *protein* for growth and for repair of the body; *minerals* and *vitamins* for growth and to keep the body functioning properly; *fat* and *carbohydrates* for energy.

Most foods contain more than one nutrient. But no single food contains all the nutrients in the amounts we need.

97

Therefore, choosing foods wisely means selecting kinds that together supply nutrients in the amounts needed. Select the main part of your diet from the four broad food groups, and try to have some meat, poultry, fish, eggs, or milk at each meal.

Milk Group

Milk is the leading source of calcium, which is needed for bones and teeth. It also provides high quality protein, riboflavin, vitamin A and many other nutrients. It may be fluid whole, evaporated, skimmed, dried, or buttermilk. Children under nine should have 2 to 3 cups daily; children nine to twelve, 3 or more cups; teen-agers, 4 or more cups; adults, 2 or more cups; pregnant women and nursing mothers, 3 to 4 cups.

Ice cream and cheese—cottage, cream or cheddar type, natural or processed—may replace part of the milk requirement. The amount needed to replace a given amount of milk is figured on the basis of calcium content. Common equivalents are: one-inch cube of cheddar-type cheese equals one-half cup of milk; one-half cup of cottage cheese equals one-third cup of milk; two tablespoons of cream cheese equal one tablespoon of milk; one-half cup of ice cream equals one-fourth cup of milk.

Meat Group

Foods in this group are valued for their protein, which is needed for growth and repair of body tissues—muscle, organs, blood, skin and hair. These foods also provide iron, thiamine, riboflavin, and niacin. Included in the group are: beef, veal, pork; variety meats such as liver, heart, kidney; poultry and eggs; fish and shellfish; and, as alternates, dry beans, dry peas, lentils, nuts, peanuts, peanut butter.

Two or more servings every day should be chosen from this group. Typical servings include: two to three ounces of lean cooked meat, poultry, or fish—all without bone; two eggs; one cup of cooked dry beans, dry peas or lentils; four tablespoons of peanut butter.

Bread-Cereal Group

This group includes all breads and cereals that are wholegrain, enriched, or restored; check labels to be sure. Among the foods in this group are breads, cooked cereals, ready-to-eat cereals, cornmeal, crackers, flour, grits, macaroni and spaghetti, noodles, rice, rolled oats and quick breads and other baked goods made with wholegrain or enriched flour. Parboiled rice and wheat also may be included in this group. These foods furnish worthwhile amounts of protein, iron, several of the B vitamins, and food energy.

Choose four or more servings daily. If no cereals are chosen, have an extra serving of breads or baked goods, which will make at least five servings from this group daily. Count as one serving: one slice of bread; one ounce of ready-to-eat cereal; one-half to three-fourths cup of cooked cereal, cornmeal, grits, macaroni, noodles, rice or spaghetti.

Vegetable-Fruit Group

All vegetables and fruits are included in this group, but their value as sources of vitamins and minerals varies considerably.

Good sources of vitamin C include grapefruit or grapefruit juice, orange or orange juice, cantaloupe, guava, mango, papaya, raw strawberries, broccoli, brussels sprouts, green pepper, sweet red pepper. Fair sources of vitamin C include honeydew melon, lemon, tangerine, watermelon, asparagus tips, raw cabbage, collards, garden cress, kale, mustard greens, potatoes and sweet potatoes cooked in the jacket, spinach, tomatoes or tomato juice, turnip greens.

Vitamin A is obtained from dark green and deep yellow vegetables and a few fruits—namely, apricots, broccoli, cantaloupe, carrots, chard, collards, cress, kale, mango, persimmon, pumpkin, spinach, sweet potatoes, turnip greens and other dark green leaves, winter squash.

Fruits and vegetables are valuable chiefly because of the vitamins and minerals they contain. This group is counted on to supply nearly all of the vitamin C needed and over half of the vitamin A. Vitamin C is needed for healthy gums and body tissues, vitamin A for growth, normal vision, and healthy condition of skin and other body surfaces.

Choose four or more servings of fruits and vegetables every day. Include one serving of a good source of vitamin C or two servings of a fair source, and one serving, at least every other day, of a good source of vitamin A. If the food chosen for vitamin C is also a good source of vitamin A, the additional serving of a vitamin A food may be omitted. The remaining one to three or more servings may be of any vegetable or fruit, including those that are valuable for vitamins C and A. Count as one serving: one-half cup of vegetable or fruit; or one medium apple, banana, orange, half a grapefruit, or juice of one lemon.

To round out meals and meet energy needs, almost everyone will use some foods not specified in the four food groups. Such foods include unenriched, refined breads, cereals and flours; sugars; butter, margarine, other fats. These often are ingredients in a recipe or are added to other foods during preparation or at the table. Try to include some vegetable oil among the fats used.

If you do not have hypoglycemia, a well-rounded diet still is essential to good health. In addition to nutrient values, you will require sufficient vitamins and minerals. Important vitamins other than those already mentioned and their sources are:

Vitamin B[6], in bananas, egg yolk, wholegrain cereals, dark green, leafy vegetables, muscle meats, liver, peanuts, yeast, prunes, raisins.

Vitamin B[12], in kidney, liver, milk, meat, cheeses, fish, egg.

Vitamin D, in egg yolk, saltwater fish, liver, vitamin D milk.

Folacin, in liver, dry beans, peanuts, walnuts, lentils, dark green vegetables.

Iodine, in iodized salt, seafood.

Magnesium, in bananas, dry beans, milk, wholegrain cereals, dark green vegetables, nuts, peanut butter.

Phosphorus, in cheese, wholegrain cereals, eggs, meat, milk, peanuts.

Vitamin E, in margarine, vegetable oils, salad dressing, peanuts, wholegrain cereals.

If you *do* have hypoglycemia, it is important that you have an understanding of diet requirements. Especially so, since you will be omitting many carbohydrates and relying mainly on proteins and fats for sustenance.

13

Questions and Answers

QUESTION: What are the common, and even uncommon, symptoms of low blood sugar?

ANSWER: Some patients have only one or two symptoms; others may have at least a half-dozen discomforting complaints, such as:

exhaustion	depression
irritability	vertigo
nervousness	insomnia
inner trembling	chronic anxiety
dizziness	drowsiness
faintness	"ulcer pains"
finger tremor	crying spells
mental confusion	phobias
headaches	personality change

indecision
allergic reactions
lessened sex drive
poor vision
weakness

"nervous breakdown"
palpatation
heart skips
sweating

QUESTION: Why does low blood sugar cause so many nervous symptoms, all the way from ordinary jittery feelings to unconsciousness?

ANSWER: Because the brain depends on the blood sugar for food and oxygen. While the rest of the tissues of the body can derive some of their energy from other fuel such as proteins and fat in the diet, the brain needs the presence of sufficient sugar to absorb oxygen normally. Therefore, it is especially sensitive to sugar deprivation. Such starvation is responsible for interference with the brain's normal metabolism and function, which accounts for some of the acute symptoms such as jittery feelings and unconsciousness. You can understand why untreated chronic hypoglycemia might actually cause some permanent brain damage.

QUESTION: What are the age limits for hypoglycemia?

ANSWER: There are none. Spontaneous hypoglycemia can occur in infants—sometimes in babies of diabetic mothers, at other times for no apparent reason. The diagnosis must be made early; otherwise, the infant's brain may be damaged. Some children who are mentally below par may have been undiagnosed cases of hypoglycemia when they were infants.

QUESTION: How do anxiety feelings and other forms of stress cause hypoglycemia?

ANSWER: Powerful emotional stress—anxiety, anger, depression, excitement—affect the metabolism of the endocrine glands. The pituitary, adrenals, thyroid, and other glands then produce malfunction in the central nervous system, which, in turn, affects the insulin mechanism in the pancreas.

QUESTION: If it is true that proteins are turned into sugar, too, why is a high protein diet advised in low blood sugar patients? Why don't they also aggravate hypoglycemia?

ANSWER: Proteins are absorbed more slowly than carbohydrates. They do not produce the sudden rise in blood sugar that causes a sensitive pancreas to oversecrete insulin and send the blood sugar level toppling. Proteins are a slower burning fuel and provide the body with a steadier blood sugar level (56 percent of proteins and 10 percent of fats are converted into sugar).

QUESTION: Just what are the normal fasting blood sugar figures?

ANSWER: To answer, I'd prefer to say "within the normal" range. For example, what is the normal pulse rate? Some say 70. But any doctor will tell you that 60 may be normal rate for one person, while another healthy person may have a rate of 80. In the same way, normal blood pressure varies in different individuals. So it is with blood sugar content. Some consider the normal fasting range to be from 65 to 110 milligrams of sugar per 100 milliliters of blood. Others say the range is between 70 and 120 milligrams. Any amount between these limits may be normal, although the figures vary with each individual. During the day, after food has been eaten, the blood sugar rises to around 140 milligrams per 100 milliliters of blood. When it rises to over 170, sugar may spill over into the urine. (A severe diabetic, for example, may have 300 mgs. in a fasting state.)

QUESTION: Why is coffee supposed to be so bad for patients with hypoglycemia?

ANSWER: Too many coffee breaks mean that too much caffeine is taken into the body. This caffeine stimulates the adrenàl gland to produce more hormones, which cause the liver to turn its glycogen into the blood stream as glucose. The excess sugar in the blood stimulates the islets of Langerhans to throw out more insulin, and the vicious circle begins again—too much insulin lowers the blood sugar to abnormal depths. Drinking coffee gives only a temporary lift, it leaves its aftereffects in symptoms caused by low blood sugar.

QUESTION: I still have symptoms that seem to be typical of low blood sugar, and my doctor agrees. But my blood sugar tolerance was not typical; it was borderline. What do you suggest?

ANSWER: It's possible for a laboratory to make a mistake. I would wait a few weeks and have another glucose tolerance test. But this time have identical samples of blood sent to different laboratories. Rechecking often reveals the true diagnosis.

QUESTION: What causes hypoglycemia? Is it hereditary?

ANSWER: I suppose you refer to idiopathic hypoglycemia, the most common type—also called functional. It is
not hereditary but probably the result of chronic stress and
anxiety which at last produces its effect on the autonomic
nervous system of the body—causing the pancreas to produce
too much insulin (hyperinsulinism).

Some people are endowed with physical and nervous systems that can withstand daily abnormal stresses. Others
are not. One way these systems break down is by developing
abnormally low blood sugar because of built-in constitutional
inadequacy. In some people, the thyroid overacts or under-
acts. In others, the pancreas malfunctions, causing either
diabetes mellitus or hypoglycemia (the opposite).

QUESTION: Can a person have a below-normal sugar
tolerance and yet show no symptoms?

ANSWER: Yes, it's possible. Also, some patients with
severe hypoglycemia may have only mild symptoms, and
vice versa.

QUESTION: How do persons with a flat glucose tolerance test react? (See Figure D.)

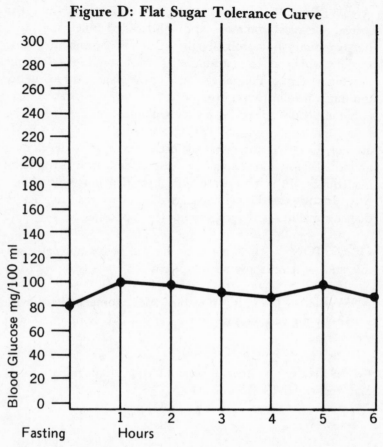

Figure D: Flat Sugar Tolerance Curve

IN THIS FLAT CURVE, NOTE THAT AFTER INGES-
TION OF SUGAR SOLUTION THE PATIENT'S BLOOD
SUGAR CONTENT DOES NOT RISE OR DROP APPRE-
CIABLY. IT REMAINS BETWEEN 80 AND 100. AL-
THOUGH IT IS NOT A TYPICAL CURVE OF HYPER-
INSULINISM, SOME PATIENTS WITH SIMILAR
CURVES COMPLAIN OF LOW BLOOD SUGAR SYMP-
TOMS.

ANSWER: Some have no symptoms at all. Others seem to be continually tired and bored. They are not fully alive. They suffer physical and emotional fatigue because their brains receive just about enough sugar to keep going rather than the normal amount necessary to live with zest and energy.

QUESTION: Is it true that diabetics are less likely to be allergic?

ANSWER: Yes, and less likely to develop rheumatic heart disease. Conversely, those with chronic low blood sugar .have a greater tendency to allergic disease and to rheumatic fever.

QUESTION: What is meant by dysinsulinism? (See Figure E.)

Figure E: Dysinsulinism

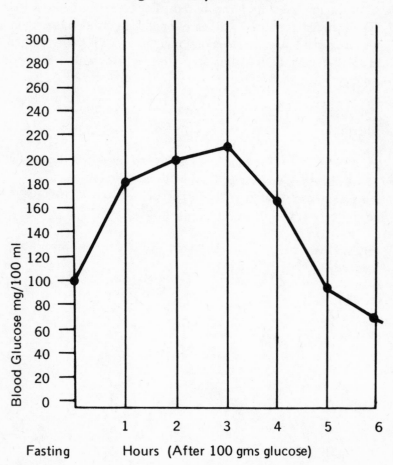

Blood Glucose mg/100 ml

Fasting   Hours (After 100 gms glucose)

A COMBINATION OF DIABETIC AND HYPOGLYCEMIC CURVES. ABOUT THREE HOURS AFTER TAKING 100 GMS. OF GLUCOSE SOLUTION, THERE IS A SHARP FALL IN BLOOD SUGAR FROM ABNORMALLY HIGH LEVELS.

ANSWER: It means that diabetes and hypoglycemia may be present at the same time. After taking sugar, the pancreas may be underactive during the first two or three hours, then become overactive (hyperinsulinism). The blood sugar drops precipitously, often causing low blood sugar symptoms in a patient who has diabetes.

QUESTION: Why do people who have low blood sugar so often become obese?

ANSWER: It is almost readily evident that they become overweight simply because they are always nibbling, but the wrong things. As the blood sugar drops, they compulsively eat sweet snacks and take sweet drinks.

QUESTION: I am forty-eight. I suppose it's the menopause, but so many complaints are blamed on the change of life, I wonder. I am nervous. I sigh a lot, more than most people. Sometimes so much that I actually shake. When a spell comes on, I get dizzy and feel faint. My heart begins to pound, and I perspire all over. Otherwise, I've been a healthy human being.

But when I get these feelings, I don't feel like any kind of human being. I get frightfully anxious that something terrible is going to happen. After a while, these scary feelings go away, and I'm able to be somewhat normal again.

Have I given you any clues? Several doctors I've seen can't find anything wrong. One says it's the menopause, and others just label my condition "nerves." Can you help? I still have a lot to live for.

ANSWER: Don't accept what I say as a definite diagnosis. It's possible that all your doctors have been correct in saying you are organically sound but suffer from nerves due to change of life. But in response to your query, "Have I given you any clues?" I can't overlook one that may be important.

I have seen a large number of patients with symptoms similar to yours who sighed a lot. Whenever I hear a nervous patient say, "I can't seem to get a full breath of air," "I'm short of breath," "I sigh a lot," then I immediately wonder if that person is suffering from unrecognized hyperventilation.

It is true that overly frequent sighing can upset the carbon dioxide-oxygen balance in the blood. Like too frequent breathing, sighing can expel too much carbon dioxide; then the chemical balance in the blood gets out of kilter. The brain, therefore, doesn't get its normal oxygen supply, and it responds by causing a variety of distressing symptoms such as sudden anxiety, heart palpitation, sweating, and dizziness.

Rebreathing into a paper bag often aborts these attacks of acute anxiety. The underlying reason, though, may be an anxiety state that requires long and patient treatment by a family doctor or by a psychiatrist. If you can learn to control your sighing, you may notice almost immediate relief. Many patients have helped themselves without depending on medical assistance.

Check on your blood sugar, too. Hypoglycemia often is associated with hyperventilation.

QUESTION: About two years ago I suffered a nervous shock caused by the unexpected death of my father. I was under a doctor's care for over a year. He gave me pills to make me less nervous.

What bothers me most lately are the awful thoughts that go through my mind. For example, if I pick up anything sharp, like a kitchen knife or large pair of scissors, I think,

"Suppose I hurt one of my children with it?" I'm a housewife and mother of 4 children, ranging in age from 18 to 21. I'm 36. Sometimes the compulsion becomes so real that I have to leave the room until it passes. I get busy doing something else to take my mind off it.

Shall I fight it alone? Do such thoughts indicate that I'm going crazy? Is there any danger?

ANSWER: I recall many patients like you. One, in particular, had similar thoughts. She had three children and would have to fight off the urge to harm them. This went on for years, but she never hurt them, nor did she ever "go crazy." About every four to six weeks she would come in to talk it over and get the "silly thoughts," as she called them, off her chest. Then she would feel better until the next time.

For months, I overlooked the possibility that hypoglycemia might be contributing to her nervousness, even though she had told me she was a poor eater. Her compulsive fears disappeared after she went on a sensible diet. Tranquilizers went into a wastebasket.

Therefore, I suggest you make an appointment for an examination. Confess your anxieties and compulsive feelings. Don't believe that your doctor will think you've been acting silly. It's not necessary to have a heart attack or broken bones in order to see him. He will give you the reassurance and medicine you need to overcome your chronic anxiety and neurosis. But insist that you will have greater peace of mind if he will send you to a laboratory for a blood sugar tolerance test. Even if it is normal, at least you will know that low blood sugar is not being overlooked.

QUESTION: I am an overweight, overworked, underpaid, nervous, tired, inefficient coffee imbiber. I have been a heavy coffee drinker for thirty years—twelve to fifteen cups a day. But I cannot break myself of the addiction. I believe it causes numbness in my extremities, nervousness, irritability, and all the other symptoms. Yet when I cut down or eliminate it, I experience headache, depression, forgetfulness, and absolute inability to function. Where do I go from here?

(I introduced her to another coffee lover. Advice coming from a layman with similar problems is often more efficacious than a lecture from a physician.)

ANSWER: First, let me explain that I'm at home all day. Without realizing it, I developed the habit of taking at least a dozen coffee breaks in addition to my usual cups at mealtime.

I never gave this a second thought until I took inventory of myself one day when I was unreasonably jittery and so tired that I could not stay awake after dinner. I made up my mind that I would limit my coffee intake to no more than two cups a day. I've been sticking to this decision for over two months now and haven't minded it a bit. I had headaches for a few days, but they disappeared. What an improvement since I cut down! I'm calmer and not tired. It's almost unbelievable.

I'm thrilled because I feel like a normal human being again. As you see, it can be done. It takes willpower, but it's worth it. I enjoy my two cups a day much more than I did when I poured it down my throat a dozen or more times a day.

(The first patient listened intently, but would she have the gumption to make the same decision?)

QUESTION: I feel I have a serious problem. I am extremely tired all the time. Some mornings I sleep until 9:30 or 10 and still find it hard to get through the day. I don't ever want to get out of bed, and when I do get up to work I feel as if it's my last day on earth—I feel so sluggish. Perhaps being the twenty-five-year-old mother of two active children, seven and five, has something to do with it.

I have been to the doctor for a physical. Everything checked out perfectly. My cholesterol is all right. I have no sugar in my urine. I have been told that I am a very nervous person, but I was never this way until lately. I'm very upset about my behavior. I feel as though I'm tranquilized by pills all the time.

Does this sound like anything serious? Is there some certain kind of test I might ask my doctor to give me? I'm scared to death.

ANSWER: Ask your doctor to have your blood sugar tested. Request a six-hour sugar tolerance curve. Anything less may not reveal the true state of affairs. Hypoglycemia may be overlooked if only a fasting blood sugar is taken, or no more than a three-hour test.

When fatigue is the presenting symptom, there are other areas of investigation. How is the function of your thyroid gland? Is it overactive? Underactive? Do you have anemia? Is your exhaustion due to emotional problems at home that you haven't mentioned? Or to some physical reason? If in doubt, ask for consultation.

QUESTION: Is or isn't there such a condition as male change of life? My friends pooh-pooh the idea.

ANSWER: I believe it is true that many men have symtoms. The condition is called the male climacteric. Most doctors share this opinion, although some still have their doubts.

There is a female menopause, or change. Men, too, are at

the mercy of their glands, although the menopause is not so dramatic in men. Some may have symptoms similar to those sometimes found in the female menopause: sweats, hot flushes, generalized weakness, lack of drive and energy, emotional instability, depression, lack of potency, and less ability to concentrate. When a woman has such symptoms while her menstrual periods are coming to an end, few doctors hesitate to say that she is in the menopause. When a man in his fifties suffers in the same way, he deserves the consideration that he, too, may need help.

Of course, the doctor should think of other possibilities as the cause of the man's symptoms: atherosclerosis of the brain arteries, psychoneurosis, or trouble due to some other organic disease. Symptoms are often so similar to those found in hypoglycemia that it is important not to overlook low blood sugar as a contributing cause of his discomfort. I have seen too many cases of male climacteric to brush aside this condition. Male hormones, too, can decline in function.

QUESTION: Why is hypoglycemia so often overlooked by physicians? (See Figure F.)

Figure F: Distortion in Sugar Curves

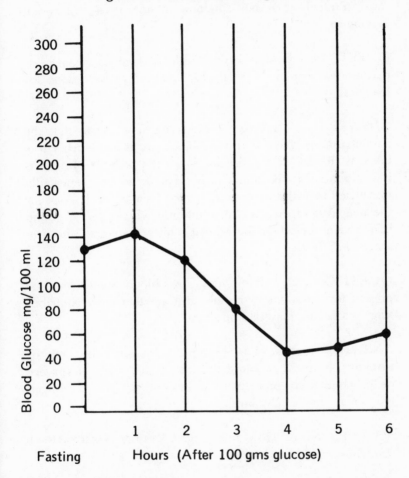

THIS READING SHOWS WHY A FASTING BLOOD SUGAR ALONE SHOULD NOT BE RELIED ON TO DE-TERMINE PRESENCE OF HYPOGLYCEMIA. IN THIS CASE, A SINGLE FASTING READING OF 130 WOULD HAVE BEEN DECEPTIVE.

ANSWER: Because most physicians are not low blood sugar minded. It is not common to find what one is not looking for.

QUESTION: Why isn't the blood sugar curve taken as part of the regular physical examination? Isn't it done for diabetes?

ANSWER: I believe the most common reason that the patient doesn't have a routine blood sugar tolerance curve taken is the doctor's desire to "save" the patient from waiting around for six hours while his veins are repeatedly punctured to withdraw blood. A blood sugar test is done for the diagnosis of diabetes mellitus only when sugar is found in the urine or when the patient's history suggests the presence of diabetes.

QUESTION: I know that low blood sugar may be present for no apparent reason. But are there any contributing factors that may be important?

ANSWER: Yes. For example, excessive smoking or drinking, frequent nibbling of sweets, the strain of surgery or of childbirth, premenstrual tension, or any prolonged emotional crisis of any kind.

QUESTION: How much sugar does the average American consume every year?

ANSWER: About 100 pounds.

QUESTION: Do you believe that anyone who has been confined as a neurotic should receive a six-hour glucose tolerance test before being discharged?

ANSWER: Yes. Many patients who discovered that they had hypoglycemia have been spared unnecessary years of mental and emotional suffering, and some, actually, from having electroshock treatments and institutional stays. Every nervous patient should have the benefit of the doubt.

QUESTION: Isn't it possible to have both a neurosis and hypoglycemia at the same time?

ANSWER: Yes. But helping the one invariably helps the other.

QUESTION: Are vitamins always necessary in treating patients who have blood sugar that is abnormally low?

ANSWER: Not always but quite often. When vitamins are deficient, there may be changes in liver function, which, in turn, disturbs carbohydrate metabolism.

QUESTION: My attacks of so-called petit mal epilepsy disappeared after the diagnosis and treatment of my low blood sugar. Is that possible?

ANSWER: Yes. There have been other instances in which hypoglycemia simulated epilepsy attacks.

QUESTION: Our marriage relationship improved after both my husband and I learned we were suffering from low blood sugar. Since we have been on our new diets, we haven't had a fight. I wonder how many marriages such a diagnosis would save?

ANSWER: To put it conservatively, thousands. I have always contended that doctors can prevent divorce. This is but one instance that proves my theory. Unhappy husbands and wives should have glucose tolerance tests.

QUESTION: My husband drinks over a dozen cups of coffee a day and at least a half-dozen cola drinks, smokes two packs, drinks a large amount of beer and whiskey, has gained much weight. But most important, he has become so irritable he's like an unlighted powder keg. I never know when he's going to explode. He refuses to go to our doctor. Do you think it's possible that he has hypoglycemia?

ANSWER: Not possible—probable.

QUESTION: Is hypoglycemia a lifelong disease?

ANSWER: In some patients, it may be a transient condition. For example, after the acute stress of an operation or after some emotional burden that lasts only for a few days or weeks. Otherwise, functional hypoglycemia may last for years.

QUESTION: In addition to diet, what drugs are used to keep the blood sugar normal?

ANSWER: When there has been a sudden drop, and blood sugar is so dangerously low as to cause convulsions or unconsciousness, injection of intravenous glucose is effective. In some cases, an injection of *glucagon* will quickly release stored glycogen from the liver into the blood stream as glucose.

Most doctors agree that tranquilizers are an excellent support for patients who are undergoing psychotherapy to overcome their anxiety-producing hypoglycemia. But there is a difference of opinion about the value of *adrenal cortical extract*. Some consider this so effectual that it should not be omitted in treatment; others are not convinced that low blood sugar patients are suffering from any inadequacy in the adrenal glands. Rather than take one side or the other, I believe that an open-minded attitude on the part of the physician is better for the patient.

QUESTION: Suppose a patient has a routine blood sugar tolerance test. It dips slightly below normal; yet he feels perfectly healthy, without any symptoms whatever. What shall he do?

ANSWER: Better forget it. In the same way, symptomless hiatal hernia patients are advised to forget it when X rays indicate the presence of a small hernia that is causing no trouble; or a symtomless diverticulosis (harmless outpouches in the intestines) patient is advised to forget it.

QUESTION: What is the difference between organic and functional hypoglycemia?

ANSWER: The organic type is caused by some actual trouble in an organ of the body: a tumor in the pancreas, a diseased pituitary or adrenal gland or a defective liver.
Functional hypoglycemia, the more common type, has no specific cause. Sometimes it will be set off by hyperventilation, by alcohol, or by taking on some silly form of crash diet to reduce weight.

QUESTION: Is the diagnosis of hypoglycemia difficult?

ANSWER: A carefully detailed history of the patient's symptoms and the glucose tolerance test usually establish the diagnosis of functional hypoglycemia. But organic low blood sugar has to be considered, especially when the patient complains most before breakfast or hours after last taking food. At such times, the question arises: Is the low blood sugar due to an insulinoma (tumor in the pancreas)? To establish the presence or absence of this organic involvement, special blood sugar studies are made after an injection of a drug called tolbutamide. A sudden sharp drop in blood sugar denotes the presence of such a tumor. Doctors will choose either surgery or medical treatment.

QUESTION: Can drinking alcohol on an empty stomach cause hypoglycemia?

ANSWER: Some people with low blood sugar are peculiarly sensitive to the effects of alcohol, especially on an empty stomach. In some cases, such a person may, after only a drink or two, act like one who is drunk. If you are suspicious about a person who has passed out without drinking heavily, consider the possibility that he has hypoglycemia. Give him orange juice to bring him around. If juice doesn't help, better call a doctor. Moral: A cocktail party is for eating as well as for drinking.

QUESTION: I have arthritis for which I take at least ten aspirin tablets a day. Lately I have noticed that I get weak feelings, perspire, and almost faint in midafternoons. My doctor ordered a blood sugar tolerance test. He says I have low blood sugar and had better cut out the aspirin. He says he will prescribe something else for the arthritis. What's wrong with aspirin?

ANSWER: There's nothing wrong with this invaluable drug. I'm sure your doctor would let you continue taking it if he hadn't found that you have low blood sugar. In some cases, there seems to be some relationship between taking aspirin and having hypoglycemia. Some hypoglycemic patients are similarly sensitive to antihistamine drugs and to barbiturates.

As you can see, the management of hypoglycemia is not a simple formula. Each patient must be studied as an individual in his responses to diet and medications.

14

Noise Pollution
as a Health Hazard

MICKEY Mouse muffs? Most visitors to an airport have seen these large protective earpieces on ground crews around jet planes. According to recent studies, noise is as much a problem in ordinary life inside or outside the home as it is around an ear-piercing jet. In fact, Dr. Austin Henschel, of Cincinnati, has said, "Potentially, the health hazard of noise is as serious as that posed by polluted air or water."

Without question, increasing noise in modern life is a serious problem. It can damage the cochlea, that part of the ear that transmits sound waves into nerve impulses. Former Surgeon General William J. Stewart of the U. S. Public Health Service even wondered if noise might not cause ulcers, mental illness, or circulation problems.

What is noise? It has been described as a meaningless pattern of sound. (Even patterned sound can be noise for the

125

especially sensitive.) The decibel, or db, is the measuring unit of sound. Two examples of varying levels of noise are the inside of a car in city traffic, which can be 85 db or more, and a New York 'subway, which is about 100 db.

But you are not free from noise in your home. The kitchen can be as noisy as the subway; the db there rises to 100 when the garbage disposal, fan, dishwasher and other electrically generated appliances all are working in concert. Of course, there is good reason for personnel to wear Mickey Mouse ear protectors when around jets, which produce 160 db.

According to an article in *Modern Medicine*, engineers consider noise levels of more than 85 db to be excessive and those over 100 db to be a cause of actual physical discomfort. For many who are supersensitive, noise is really a form of torture (as in a case history I shall relate later).

Even teenagers are in danger of losing their hearing perceptivity, according to some recent observations. According to Dr. Charles P. Lebo, of the University of California, background noise levels in full-volume discotheques often reach peaks of 120 db. If a teenager is exposed to these levels for four hours a day, two days per week, and continues this exposure rate for a year or more, there is likely to be some permanent hearing loss. This permanent hearing loss is comparable to the neural deafness found in the elderly.

Although I agree that there is need for continued study to determine if noise is as great a threat as it seems to be, I recognize that the pendulum has a tendency to swing too widely whenever any new theory is advanced. There are two sides. I like to consider the moderate approach, too.

For example, consider this statement by Dr. Leo Beranek of the acoustics firm of Bolt, Beranek, and Newman:

The noises of our daily life have been blamed variously for the high divorce rate, social conflict, indigestion and other organic disabilities, nervous breakdown, high blood pressure, heart failure, and even insanity.

Most of these allegations arise from over-vivid imaginations. Still one cannot completely rule out the possibility that some people are particularly sensitive to noise just as others are allergic to nuts, eggs, or household dust.

Earlier I mentioned the case history of an extremely noise-sensitive person. Here it is.

"For the past ten months I have been going out of my mind because of a television set my downstairs neighbors bought last fall. They like their noise loud, but I am getting the bass tones and the vibrations from this set. They do not hear what I have to hear.

"I have run out of this apartment in tears night after night. I have had to seek refuge with a neighbor until these people went to bed. I would be in a panic up here, pacing back and forth and having palpitations so bad that I thought I was having a heart attack. Why didn't I complain? I have. But it didn't help. The husband said his wife had a stroke some years ago, her TV set is her only amusement.

"The culmination of all this mess is that I can't keep up in my business in my present state. My nerve panic has carried over. To make it worse, I had renewed my lease just before they bought this set. I have been trapped.

"These people just can't understand. They imply that I am a miserable person, depriving this woman of her only pleasure in life. They kept the sound down for a week, but now it's up full force again.

"This whole thing has become psychologically bad for me. I can't keep fighting a handicapped woman. But since I've been home for a few weeks because of illness, I have to listen to twelve to fifteen hours of TV blasting every day. I'm flying apart. I cannot stand this. Now I'm in such a state that everytime the TV goes on I dread the day, I'm so apprehensive. As I said, I have to get out of here , but I'm trapped."

I cannot recall ever having seen a more miserable looking patient. She was completely exhausted and enervated. She begged me to do something that might help.

In questioning her, I found that she had overlooked some practical aids. I prescribed tranquilizers and occasional sleeping pills to overcome or neutralize her nervousness and insomnia. (Previously, she could not be convinced to take "dope.") I suggested she buy some ear plugs. ("Now why didn't I think of those?" she said). She also gave a history of having lost weight because "I've been so nervous I haven't been eating sensibly. Just been nibbling on bread and butter, filling up on candies and cookies—too tired and nervous to make myself a good meal at night."

The ridiculously happy ending to this "horror story" came about after a blood sugar tolerance test showed that she had also been suffering from low blood sugar. (To theorize, the constant noise had overstimulated her adrenal glands, which, in turn, had overstimulated her pancreas and caused hyperinsulinism).

She went on a high protein, low carbohydrate diet, eating six meals daily. Within a week, she had been transformed into a quiet, understanding person. In fact, she now visited her neighbor often to bring her comfort. Their television set no longer bothered her. Had they cut down the volume? "I really haven't noticed," she said.

Learning to Live with Noise

More and more people are complaining about noise. They say they are very sensitive to it. What can they do about a noisy neighbor or some other distraction? I tell them that noise is an integral part of the twentieth-century life, but that even our forebears had the rumble of occasional thunder to contend with. We must learn to live with, and protect ourselves against, the daily thunder of the jets, not to mention scores of other noises that are a part of this machine age. And we must not blame it all on machines.

Practical philosophy helps us to bear it. For example, our next door neighbor's little son is learning how to play the trumpet. I admire his tenacity but deplore the sounds that come from his desire to learn. Yet after hearing a few blasts, I begin to philosophize—and the little fellow's practicing session is over before I realize it. All I have to do to bear it is to think of the scratchy, unbearable whines that struggled forth from my fiddle when I practiced as a youngster. There were no tranquilizers for neighbors in those days. No theories that an abnormally low blood sugar might be intensifying the discomforts.

Recently a woman asked, "How do you feel about noise? Can't it make people sick? As for myself, I've gotten so I can't stand any kind of noise: children playing, brakes screeching or even someone turning the page of a book. What's the answer?"

I told her that while she continued to live in this increasingly noisy century she had better find some way to get used to it, or it would actually make her sick—psychologically as well as physically. Loss of hearing isn't the only bad potential effect.

I agree that repeated exposure to the intense noise of a jet engine, for example, might cause hearing trouble. But when the pages of a book being turned cause distress, then I'd rate the trouble as being psychological as well as physical.

I have known several patients who have been especially noise-sensitive. When nothing else helped, I was sure to check on their blood sugar. If that was all right, and nothing else seemed to help, I have used shock therapy in word form to immunize them against their reaction to noise. At first, they recoiled from it, but later they admitted that it produced remarkable improvement.

I say to them, "See if you can project yourself far enough into the future to imagine yourself no longer a member of this earthly planet. Can you feel the stillness, the unwelcome, unbroken quiet? Not even the chirping of birds in a world silent and devoid of all noise? Imagine that distant day when all will be quiet. Wouldn't you give anything to be able to hear again the squeals of children, brakes screeching, the turn of a page? Think of this the next time you become upset by noise. Within seconds, you will dismiss any annoyance and replace it with a feeling of thankfulness that you are still around to enjoy sounds, whatever they are."

I have come across an interesting script produced for radio presentation by Charles Levy and William Howe for the University of California. It is called "Noise Unlimited." They mention that scientists have found an apt phrase to describe the ever-increasing environmental cacophony. They call it audio pollution (sister to air, water, and soil pollution).

For example, in a recent study of the residents of Caracas, Venezuela, a group of professors report, "It's the terrible noise that has turned citizens from happy, friendly people into grouchy persons who generally also suffer from poor hearing. Factory noises, cars, and motorcycles without mufflers, police whistles and juke boxes make life miserable here."

According to Dr. Walter W. Soroka, professor of acoustical sciences of the University of California:

> There's still a good deal of controversy regarding the health aspects of noise, and so far very little positive information has been made available through medical research.
>
> One difficult aspect of this whole question is that people do become adapted to noise if they live with it long enough. It is only when the noise changes to an increased level, well above the level to which they've been accustomed, that they begin to fret about it. And if nothing is done, they'll get used to that too.

I'm sure he doesn't mean you'll get used to standing by a revved up jet engine, and neither do I. But I think that an acceptance of the ordinary noises (not physically harmful) that upset some people so much is possible by a new psychological approach. Why not try the shock treatment I have recommended? If you have a vivid imagination, it will quickly wipe out any irritations you may suffer at present.

And do not overlook the possibility that protracted noises may have had some effect on the adrenals and indirectly on the pancreas and insulin secretion. In laboratory experiments on mice, for example, exposure to high-pitched sounds has produced convulsions. Yet these seizures diminished in intensity, and at last gradually disappeared, when they were given more adequate diets with a high vitamin content.

Although human beings do not ordinarily go into convulsive seizures because of diet or vitamin deficiency when exposed to the daily stress of noise, the consideration of possible hypoglycemia is not invariably a far-fetched theory. Low blood sugar can intensify and cause distress, whatever the source of stress.

15

Jungle Anxieties
in Civilized Man

Some time ago I saw a Walt Disney motion pic-
ture called *Nature's Half-Acre*. It is an interesting portrayal
of teeming life and sudden death. It shows nature as interested only in preserving the species, not the individual.
There are beautiful representations of the four seasons,
which to the imagination readily recall infancy, adolescence,
maturity, and old age.

As you watch, entranced, you realize there really is no
basic distinction between "upper" and "lower" life. All life stems
from the same mysterious source and ends in an equally unknown destination. You can learn much about life if you are
in the mood to absorb the picture fully.

You see the ravenously hungry caterpillars, who are
grossly fat—fatter than pigs. How persistently they gnaw the
leaves. They are in a great hurry to enjoy, because they

133

seem to sense doom surely settling down on them. And it is, for next you are shown a nest with four hungry throats wide open, spread by sharp beaks. And you see the mother bird looking down into the nest and catching on to what the commotion is all about. They are starved. She flies like a shot from the nest, and you know it is doomsday for the caterpillar. When we observe him next, he is being forced down the willing throat of a hungry baby bird.

Incidentally, closely examine the countenance—if you can call it that—of the baby bird as he impatiently awaits his food. You never saw a more stern, angry, and demanding manner. You think of the human youngster, and forgive him his tantrums and incivility when he is hungry. You think of how low blood sugar affects the brain, and how its messages, received from an empty stomach, convert a sweet person to a temporarily sour one.

Also note that mother bird does not admonish her youngsters for lack of table manners. She seems to care only that they eat, be healthy, and survive. Growing up will take care of their manners. At least they will be free of neurosis caused by too strict supervision at breakfast, lunch, and dinner.

The little birds are hungry, and they *yell*. And they expect to be fed. They are veritable little villains. You smile as you watch, and you come to the conclusion that children are the same the world over, especially hungry children.

Throughout the motion picture, you have the feeling of life being lived intensely. There is the strong undercurrent of the struggle for survival. Of course, the fittest survived, but none is free from the danger of extinction. Even the fit fly or the strong, industrious bee is not proof against the silken chains of the spider. You see many a juicy insect rolled snugly in a web and stored away until a future appetite calls it forth again. (How now, low blood sugar?)

There are traps for ants as they work in the sand. Flies have not only spiders to contend with (and fly swatters) but also beautiful, sweet-smelling plants that entrap them and digest them.

You see horrendously shaped creatures that fight each other to the death. They are members of the same animal classification. (You think, perhaps, of the Civil War.) Imaginations need not be fertile to see the resemblance between "low life" and "high life." In fact, there is more than a resemblance: it is the same.

In high and low alike, we find passion, appetite, fear, compulsion to work and procreate and compulsion to survive. We observe cruelty, jealousy, envy and occasional lack of compassion. There is thanklessness planning for the future. The four seasons for the insects and the birds—as for us—are the magic, ever-recurring renewal of life.

You come away from the theater (if you are at all open to suggestion) with the feeling that you have been privileged to peek behind the curtain. You feel that all animals are one, that we stem from one force, that we all live in a jungle. Ours, perhaps, has been cleared away more. The stuff we call civilization has been of use in seasoning our existence; the only hope for the human is the speed with which he can deepen the very thin layer of "culture" that separates him from the lowest animals.

That speed, I think, will depend on how soon there is a truer balance between the heart and the head. So far, the human brain has outstripped the heart. When our emotions catch up with our thoughts, and vice versa, that will be the millenium.

We need to be more civilized. The animal and human jungles are too far apart. As a rule, animals fight each other only when they are hungry; men fight with their bellies full. But sometimes we are not aware that our bellies are full of the wrong kind of food. If there is a dearth of proteins and a superabundance of carbohydrates in the stomach, the brain suffers for lack of sugar, because insulin has deleted large quantities from the blood stream. We become jittery and nervous, and short-tempered. We are too ready to fight.

For self-preservation, if for no other reason, it is essential that man be aware of the need for having normal and sufficient blood sugar. Not until then can he look on the harried animals in the jungle and say, "Too bad you can't be like us."

Parting Note

I'll probably never know how many readers of this book have suffered (or are still suffering) from what they have believed to be a hapless "nervousness" for which there is no relief.

I make this request: whoever or whatever you are, please do not procrastinate. Ask your physician to arrange for a complete blood sugar study. Too many live half a life simply because they are unaware that they are sugar-starved.

Hopelessness feeds on one's lack of effort to help oneself. More than you realize, your life is in your own hands.

137

Index

O

Obesity, 111
  and compulsive eating, 40, 41
  and duodenal ulcer, 79-80
  eating habits causing, 39
Overwork, and fatigue, 29

P

Pancreas, 19-24
  anatomy, 20
  blocking of insulin secretion, 24, 93
  in control of sugar metabolism, 22
  effect of noise on, 128, 131
  insulin production affected by stress, 105, 107
  islet tumor of, 12, 122
  physiology, 20-22, 93, 106
Personality, change in, 45-52
Petit mal epilepsy
  and hypoglycemia, 119
  vs. narcolepsy, 42
Physical checkups, need for, 88-90
Pituitary gland
  blocking insulin secretion, 24
  insufficiency, 16
Polycythemia, causing fatigue, 35

R

Relaxation
  during working day, 33
  methods, 32-33
Rest
  frequent, 34
  need for, 30-33
Rheumatic fever, and sugar metabolism, 109
Rheumatic heart disease, treatment, 83
Ritalin
  to combat narcolepsy, 39, 41, 42
  in test for narcolepsy, 43
Road hypnosis, 38

S

Sleep, lack of, and fatigue, 29
Sleepiness. *See* Narcolepsy
Smoking
  effect on blood sugar, 14
  effect on heart, 73
  and fatigue, 29
Snacks, between-meal, 14
Social drinkers, 85
Stress, effects of, 105, 107
Sugar
  abnormal metabolism, 22-23
  consumption in America, 118